COVID 19:
A Pandemic of Ignorance, Fear, Hysteria and "Official Truth" Lies

James DeMeo, PhD

COVID 19:
A Pandemic of Ignorance, Fear, Hysteria and "Official Truth" Lies

James DeMeo, PhD

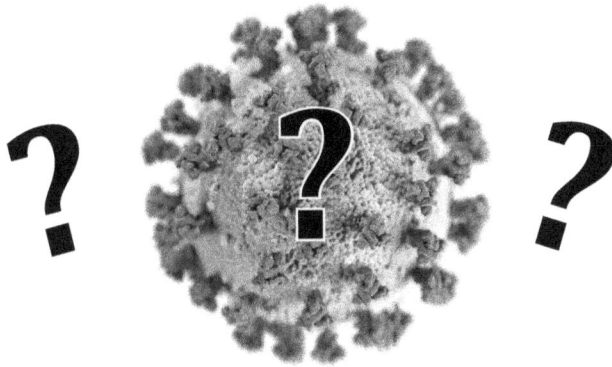

An independent scientific review fails to confirm the central claims of the CDC, WHO, NIH, FDA, alarmist media & political tyrants

Updated Sept. 2021
Natural Energy Works
Ashland, Oregon, USA
www.naturalenergyworks.net

World-wide Publication and Distribution:

Natural Energy Works
PO Box 1148
Ashland, Oregon 97520
United States of America
www.naturalenergyworks.net
info@naturalenergyworks.net

ISBN: 978-0-9974057-5-0

This book is an expanded version of a prior research article by James DeMeo entitled *A Critical Review of CDC USA Data on Covid-19: PCR/Antigen Tests & Cases Reveal Herd Immunity Only, and Do Not Warrant Public Hysteria or Lockdowns.*

20210914

Front Cover virus image, and electron micrograph images elsewhere, courtesy of NIH/CDC/NIAID. Figures 1-6 and 9 graphics, courtesy of the Our World in Data group, reproduced in color on the inside covers.

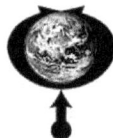

"Unless we put medical freedom into the Constitution, the time will come when medicine will organize into an undercover dictatorship... To restrict the art of healing to one class of men and deny equal privileges to others will constitute the Bastille of medical science. All such laws are un-American and despotic and have no place in a republic... The Constitution of this Republic should make special privilege for medical freedom as well as religious freedom."

- Benjamin Rush, MD, c.1789

Signer of the *Declaration of Independence,*
Physician to George Washington,
From *The Autobiography of Benjamin Rush*

Chapter Sections

Page

Author's Acknowledgements

My thanks to all those who gave helpful advice and constructive critical review of my manuscript, for this book as well as for the summary article that preceded it. Especially I wish to thank my wife Daniela Bruckner, and good friends Thomas DiFerdinando and Ira Bauer, for proof-reading and constructive scientific critique. Very much appreciated. J.D.

"What is the hardest thing of all?
That which seems the easiest.
For your eyes to see,
that which lies before your eyes."
– Goethe

Preface

This is a book I never intended to write. Its origin was my own outrage about the deadly ignorance, hysteria and lies that permeate the claims about an alleged SARS-CoV-2 virus causing a new disease "Covid-19". My expertise in both the physical and natural sciences, with considerable prior work on health-related issues, and as a long-time critic of mainstream allopathic pharmacy-driven medicine, also demanded this book.

The basic structure of our constitutional Republic has been warped, forced to conform to the totalitarian demands of a claimed infectious Covid-19 viral pandemic. Investigating, I found serious problems in logic and causality, with a reckless abuse of data by professionals and journalists, whose job is to safeguard the facts, and public health. They let everyone down. The fingerprints of the Chinese Communist Party also became clear, conspiring with American medicine and pharmaceutical interests, and with communists in positions of power at the highest levels. One is reminded of the 20th Century debacles of Lysenko, Mengele, the euthanasia and eugenics experiments, all of which were supported by "top" people, with widespread censorship and punishment of dissent. Covid-19 similarly carries an entire raft of mass-psychological social terrorism, in which allopathic medicine, the radical Left media and power-drunk collectivist politicians have all exerted a deadly influence.

I began writing on the Covid-19 subject starting in mid-2020, when the outlines of the catastrophes of error and deception became clear. I made my own analysis of official data sources regarding Covid-19, and later of the VAERS vaccine death and injury data. A preliminary article was written in January 2021,[‡] and widely circulated on internet, obtaining informal peer-review with periodic updates. That article is now incorporated into this book, with much newly-added material.

Here, I raise an alarm, about the deadly errors and deception at work within our science, public health and political institutions. Many brave and honest physicians and scientists have already spoken out in dissent, and paid a heavy price for doing so. They should not stand alone, and once more, I add my voice to the chorus of dissent.

– James DeMeo, PhD, June 2021
Ashland, Oregon, USA

‡ DeMeo J: A Critical Review of CDC USA Data on Covid-19: PCR/Antigen Tests & Cases Reveal Herd Immunity Only, and Do Not Warrant Public Hysteria or Lockdowns. www.researchgate.net/publication/348550612

Introduction

Were we deceived? Are we still? Was the entire "Covid-19" program one Big Lie? A con-job aimed at empowering already power-drunk and profiteering political, medical and "health care" bureaucracies, and their pharmaceutical company bosses? A shell-game in which predominantly elderly people above the ages of 65, already suffering from multiple crippling comorbidities, were ushered into an early grave by malignant hospital care and denial of inexpensive and effective medicines? Was it a true "viral pandemic", or a pandemic of ignorance, panic, hysteria and "official truth" lies? Are we continuing to be deceived, for the next "virus variant", the next "pandemic", to shield those with blood on their hands? And what about the massive censorship? The cover-up of crimes committed by leading Covid "authorities"? The silencing of brave doctors, scientists and journalists who dare to speak truth to the power-drunk? The citizens who refuse to mask, dare to keep open a business which is their own thin lifeline of survival, the preachers who dare to open up a church, those who walk alone on a beach without a mask, they were and are punished severely, often with thousands in fines and jail time. Should we just shrug it off? Do nothing? Ignore what happened, including the economic devastation demanded by "top" medical and political authorities with financial and ideological ties to foreign despots?

Around a half-million Americans were sent to early graves due to Covid, according to the latest statistics. Should we just ignore that, bury grandma and grandpa, or parents and friends, and forget what happened? Blame "the virus", ignore the human role, and also not look in the mirror? Ignore the power-drunk governors who issued arbitrary unconstitutional edicts? Ignore the correlated crooking of elections in November 2020, facilitated by lockdown and distancing rules where oversight was rendered impossible? How many other social institutions were converted during Covid into instruments of deception and oppression? How many people and communities were driven over the edge into catastrophic situations due to the indefensible claims by a small number of compromised scientists and physicians, helped along by crooked mainstream media and the censorious totalitarian behavior of internet billionaires?

There are many questions needing clear answers, even as this claimed "viral pandemic" is winding down. Or is that yet another deception? Consider the following critical factors and evidence which, among others, are detailed in this book.

Firstly, what is a "pandemic"? Dating back at least to February 2003, the World Health Organization (WHO) defined "pandemic" accurately, within the context of recurring bouts of influenza:

> "An influenza pandemic occurs when a new influenza virus appears against which the human population has no immunity, resulting in several, simultaneous epidemics worldwide *with enormous numbers of deaths and illness*."[1] (emphasis added)

That was a rational definition, indicating a multi-regional *pandemic* of high death tolls was far worse than a more regionally isolated *epidemic* of merely spreading infections and fewer deaths. In September 2009, however, the pandemic definition was radically changed, removing the specific language regarding "enormous numbers of deaths and illness". The new definition was vague enough to apply in a wide variety of circumstances: "A disease epidemic occurs when there are more cases of that disease than normal. A pandemic is a worldwide epidemic of a disease."[2] WHO stated this change in definition would allow for a more rapid response to *presumed forthcoming pandemics* of infectious and deadly disorders, predominantly for development of vaccines and other pharmaceutical drugs.

That was during a growing outbreak of "virus H1N1 influenza A variant", also called the Swine Flu, where cases were determined by both the inaccurate Polymerase Chain Reaction (PCR) lab-test, and the more subjective clinical presentation of symptoms. Swine Flu was then declared a "pandemic" without the previously required "enormous numbers of deaths". But the new criteria thereafter became generally mixed up with less deadly "epidemics" of ordinary influenza or Severe Acute Respiratory Syndrome (SARS). Strains of Avian Flu, Hong Kong Flu, Swine Flu, Middle East Respiratory Syndrome (MERS) and others received, by my observation, ambiguous classifications as either epidemics or pandemics. According to their symptoms, all were SARS-like influenza, with questionable viral causations and rushed vaccination programs. Global infections with massive death-counts were no longer necessary.

An interesting comparison is that the same 2009 Swine Flu "H1N1 Influenza A" variant was previously identified in an early 1976 outbreak, for which a vaccine was rushed into production within three months. That vaccination program was halted after 54 people died from its side-effects, specifically from the rare auto-immune disorder Guillain-Barré syndrome, resulting in respiratory distress and paralysis.[3]

Almost one year after the WHO changed the pandemic definition, in May 2010, the Rockefeller Foundation (RF) – a long-time supporter of allopathic medicine and pharmaceutical drugs – published "Scenarios for the Future of Technology and International Development".[4] This document speculated what action should be taken in the event of infectious pandemics over the next 15 years, suggesting lockdowns, forced masking, isolations, loss of freedoms and other draconian measures would be necessary. Ten years hence, their "fictional supposition" was finally realized with Covid-19.[4]

In November of 2019, just prior to the announcement of SARS-CoV-2 and Covid-19 disease, WHO also revised its *pandemic guidelines*, which over decades had declared *against* widespread forced lockdowns of asymptomatic populations, forced masking and inhuman isolation.[5] (see Figure 12, page 45). For Covid-19, and for the first time in the history of public health, all such draconian dictates once termed "not recommended under any circumstance" by old-school physicians and epidemiologists, were now deemed "acceptable" *for entire nations!*

By late January 2020, a report by Corman-Drosten, et al. was published claiming the development of a PCR test for SARS-CoV-2.[6] However, these claims were not based upon isolated DNA sequences of living virus, but were *artificially created by sheer speculations typed into a computer* ("in silico"!). This guaranteed the new tests would yield erroneous cross-reactivity with all kinds of unknown RNA-DNA material from multiple microbial, viral and cellular break-down fragments. Such cellular debris is commonly found among human populations exposed over years to ordinary colds and influenza. Corman-Drosten et al. admitted "virus isolates are unavailable" but claimed *the specific SARS-CoV-2 virus material did not have to be present in the development of their PCR tests for them to work*. They wrote: "We aimed to develop and deploy robust diagnostic methodology for use in public health laboratory settings without having virus material available."[6] Stunningly, this paper was roundly applauded by mainstream science and medicine as "proof" for PCR identification of SARS-CoV-2. High rates of false positives were anticipated by professional critics of their paper, who called for its retraction.[7] Such scientific dissent and challenges were ignored, however, and the Corman-Drosten et al. PCR testing methods were rushed into mass production.

In February 2020, as the Covid-19 disaster was emerging, the US Centers for Disease Control (CDC) similarly exercised its muscle to *change the methods of disease data collection and counting*, allowing for a sloppy mix of methods such as unreliable PCR tests, antigen tests, and subjective clinical diagnoses to define cases and deaths from "Covid-19", even if they otherwise appeared to be ordinary influenza or other known lung disorders.[8] In doing so, the CDC thereby abandoned a proven prior method they had successfully employed nationwide since 2003. Following that change, they reported the numbers of Covid-19 "infections" had swelled, even as influenza "inexplicably" declined (see Figures 7 and 8, page 31).

Adding scientific insult to medical injury, the WHO also re-defined the long established meaning of *herd immunity* for the Covid-19 "pandemic". By the old definition, survival and recovery from natural infections or exposures was the primary path to both individual and herd immunity, whether or not one got sick or remained asymptomatic and healthy. As recently as late October 2020, the WHO had declared:

> "Herd immunity is the indirect protection from an infectious disease that happens when a population is immune either through vaccination *or immunity developed through previous infection.*"[9] (emphasis added)

The older definition acknowledged how humans could be exposed to and survive a host of lesser infectious diseases, acquiring natural immunity individually, or herd immunity collectively, without use of vaccines. And indeed, from October through December 2020, astonishing numbers of Americans "tested positive" but remained asymptomatic, *indicating herd immunity had already been acquired.* However, starting in early November and in anticipation of massive international vaccine programs, the WHO ignored such clear evidence, and *deleted all mention of natural immune responses to infection from its public notices, as if they did not exist!*

> "'Herd immunity', also known as 'population immunity', is *a concept used for vaccination, in which a population can be protected from a certain virus if a threshold of vaccination is reached. Herd immunity is achieved by protecting people from a virus, not by exposing them to it.*"[10] (emphasis added)

This was a clear example of growing scientism and medical fraud favoring expensive pharmaceutical remedies, and not for the first or last time. Naturally acquired herd immunity was declared as a mere "concept", and subordinated to the application of vaccinations. Medical "experts" had already been denouncing the use of effective and inexpensive medicines such as hydroxychloroquine, ivermectin, zinc, vitamins C and D in higher doses, and any other kind of non-pharmaceutical approach that would keep people out of the hospitals and make vaccinations unnecessary. Research studies proving the efficacy of the older remedies were suppressed by the mainstream media and internet billionaires, as were the physicians who used them to cure their patients. Medical and media alarmism made people afraid to treat their cold or flu symptoms by ordinary bed-rest, vitamins, herbal teas or grandma's garlic-chicken soup (a marvelous immune-boosting remedy). Public paranoia emerged about unmasked faces, and even unmasked family and friends. Lockdowns, masking and vaccines were the only way to halt the pandemic, it was claimed. Most people obeyed, in fear, or with "heroic" boasting vainglory. By 2021, populations lined up in droves for the medical Holy Waters.

The public health was thereafter placed at the mercies of profiteering pharmaceutical firms devoted to vaccinations as the only possible remedy for infectious disorders. At present, the "officially declared" USA threshold for herd-immunity claims 70% of the population must be vaccinated, no matter how many recovered from Covid-19 or remained asymptomatic. As noted in an ending chapter, it seems unlikely that more than around half the USA population will take the vaccines, largely due to the high numbers of deaths they have already caused – over 5000 dead by mid-June 2021, but no outcry from the medical community (as with Swine Flu deaths, to halt their use). Despot politicians are now pushing "vaccine passports", or extended lockdowns to punish the educated disobedient.

Humanity overcame Swine Flu, in both 1976 and 2009, and all other infectious disorders since, primarily by achieving natural herd immune system responses to them. And we did so, repeatedly, with little or no vaccination interventions of significance – until Covid 19, when the fraudulent re-definitions by the WHO, CDC, and the National Institutes of Health (NIH) declared otherwise. The US Food and Drug Administration (FDA) also played its deadly role by granting "emergency authorization" of experimental antiviral drugs and mRNA vaccines, whose toxic side-effects were better documented than their claimed protective magic.

The ability of the conventional-thinking and financially-compromised global health bureaucracy to re-define "pandemic" and "herd immunity" by mere declaration was significant, as it granted them the power to exert control over the situation – the facts, truth and public health be damned. These events of 2020 were also conditioned by earlier schemes and plots initiated at the highest levels of international politics.

There was the October 2019 "Event 201 Pandemic Exercise" organized by the World Economic Forum (WEF) and the Bill and Melinda Gates Foundation (GF).[11] This meeting included the virology bureaucrats, pharmaceutical cartels, representatives of WHO, CDC, NIH, FDA and other globalist representatives from around the world, laying out a hypothetical situation of a major coronavirus outbreak, and how best to handle it (with draconian lockdown measures and vaccines). It was a "fictional scenario", we were told. But, was it?

Shortly thereafter came the deceptive and alarming behavior of the Communist Chinese at the Wuhan Virology Institute, firstly in their denial of "gain of function research" (ie, making a benign virus deadly) and secondly by accidentally or deliberately allowing a claimed "weaponized" bat-virus to escape into the local communities, frightening the Chinese citizens into a panic. Draconian lockdowns followed and the entire city of Wuhan was quarantined for months. Soon after, the WHO recommended the entire world follow the "Chinese Model" of virus containment, even though by independent analysis, this new alleged virus *wasn't causing mass deaths*, even if public media announcements suggested otherwise. Mass fear and panic ensued. Was that the goal?

Then there was the admission by top world leaders to openly abuse the "Covid-19 pandemic" to bring about long-cherished globalist "New World Order" changes, as found in the alarming book *Covid-19: The Great Reset* by Klaus Schwab.[12] Schwab was the founder of the WEF, an anti-freedom insiders club of proto-communist corporate billionaires and their media, medical and political camp followers. The same "Great Reset" was adopted as a WEF conference theme in June 2020.[13] These new anti-freedom social forces openly applauded the Covid-19 "economic restructuring" (lockdown destruction of small-business capitalism, enriching global corporations) and environmental "benefits" (communist-green ideology). They advocated for continued restrictions on freedom, democracy, economies, movement and independence as a permanent and standardized way of life for all of humanity (excluding themselves, of course).

Not surprisingly, massive censorship descended upon American citizens like never before, starting in 2020 and continuing into 2021. Internet billionaires led the movement to silence and personally destroy anyone who dared to question the "official truth" about Covid-19, or who advocated for inexpensive and effective medicines that would interfere with the WHO claim that "only vaccines can stop the pandemic". Such censorship already existed on other topics (ie, forbidding criticism of "climate change" or "genderism") but was increasingly criminalized and expanded. Mainstream media also endorsed the whole basket of organized Covid-19 "official truths", skewing the news in favor of whatever the WHO, CDC, FDA, NIH, WEF, GF and RF might desire.

The average person and concerned professionals should have been alarmed by these unilateral anti-freedom and anti-science measures. Some were, but the majority were not, at least initially.

As I will demonstrate, there are gigantic errors and misrepresentations of science and medicine associated with Covid-19, going way beyond the fraudulent redefinitions of important concepts, distorting their meanings. No matter where one shines the light of scientific logic and reason within the Covid-19 universe, looking for evidence, one emerges empty-handed, and certainly no gold standard of proofs can be found by which the larger "Covid-19 pandemic" paradigm could survive. Point by point, I will examine the claimed evidence, in depth, exposing the inconsistencies, flaws and lack of clear causality.

One of the primary missions and responsibilities of the scientific world, as in the healing arts and medicine, is to make accurate observations, analyses and predictions based upon rational logic and causality. When science or medicine strays from that mission, and promotes inaccurate, or top-heavy, speculative theories for social application or government policy, the consequences are predictably disastrous. Modern medicine is not immune from such risks. A case in point are the claims about a deadly virus SARS-CoV-2 causing Covid-19 disease, even as SARS and influenza are real and potentially deadly conditions. It is the *theories about SARS and other pulmonary disorders claimed to be Covid-19, and how they are caused,* against which I raise an objection.

One of the greatest flaws and inconsistencies within the "official" Covid-19 theory or paradigm is how laboratory tests supposedly identify "cases" among predominantly asymptomatic people, but nevertheless *fails to predict* who will get sick and die, versus those who will remain healthy and live. We expect a true infectious pandemic with so many "confirmed by laboratory testing" *cases,* to predict and drive up the "confirmed *deaths* by Covid-19", in a manner far more direct and substantial than is observed. *This has not happened, even as widespread panic, fear and isolation misery pushed many elderly with multiple comorbidities into early graves.*

As another example, early in 2020, diagnoses of Covid-19 disease were made solely by clinical observations of real SARS/influenza symptoms. The diagnostic criteria included difficulty breathing, fever, chills, heavy mucous coatings in the throat and upper windpipe, a "ground glass" opacity on chest x-rays, and other pulmonary symptoms, often accompanied by heart irregularities. What formerly was diagnosed and treated as SARS/ influenza was suddenly, with the fear of a deadly super-virus escaped from Wuhan China, being identified (or misidentified) as Covid-19.

Seemingly credible reports told of massive numbers of people dying in Wuhan, with videos of panicked people overwhelming hospitals, sometimes dropping dead in the street. Panic and hysteria were created globally among the front-line nurses and doctors, and the general public. Hazmat suits, gloves, masks, isolation wards and other measures were instituted to protect hospital staff and to contain the spread of a presumed new and potentially deadly and infectious airborne virus. Patients with SARS-like symptoms, or sometimes just a cold or flu were rushed to hospitals, put into isolation wards, treated as if they had the black plague, with some placed on potentially deadly ventilators. With medical and media alarmist reporting, fear of a deadly contagion spread throughout the general population. Lockdowns were instituted to "flatten the curve" of infections, which reportedly were necessary to give hospitals time to "catch up" with the growing number of claimed-Covid-19 infections. One excuse after another was then offered up to make the lockdowns permanent. Most people did not question "medical authority", and the crisis triggered opportunistic or pre-planned totalitarian political reactions.

Panic and anxiety added to physical distress, especially as elderly people with pre-existing respiratory symptoms were given a Covid-19 diagnosis, with similar questionable treatments. *This is what drove up the death numbers, as I will demonstrate.* There has been a general failure among all parties – medicine, science, media and government – to appreciate that fact and to remain open to other causes.

Whether or not these steps were justified, deaths increased, particularly among elderly populations who sought refuge or treatment in the hospitals, and many more died in nursing homes where isolation from loved ones, anxiety and suffering were amplified. Some states like New York transferred sick elderly people from hospitals into nursing homes, where hospital-like containment of their many comorbidities was impossible, and deaths soared. The issue of whether these people were suffering from a new disease (Covid-19) created by an infectious new virus, or merely from ordinary lung and heart disorders, with similar presenting symptoms, remained an open question rarely asked. In early 2020, I had no reason to seriously question the official narratives about Covid-19, but became increasingly skeptical, for the reasons which follow.

PCR/Antigen Confirmed "Cases"
Do Not Support a Claimed "Pandemic"

By March of 2020, new forms of laboratory test diagnosis for claimed SARS-CoV-2 became widely available, such as Polymerase Chain Reaction (PCR) biochemical tests (discussed in detail in a separate section). Additional antigen tests were also subsequently developed, and today there is a wide range of PCR/Antigen testing devices. These tests were claimed to produce more accurate diagnosis of Covid-19 than could be obtained by clinical diagnosis of presenting symptoms only. However, both the PCR and antigen tests were over-hyped, and never so accurate in their determinations. A comparison of the claimed "laboratory confirmed" cases and deaths reveal this to be true.

Data on the Covid-19 numbers, such as "confirmed cases" and "confirmed deaths" were firstly tracked on a weekly basis and published in early May of 2020 by the US Center for Disease Control (CDC). I watched those numbers steadily grow, but found a more reliable graphic presentation of the *daily* data reports at the *Our World In Data (OWID)* website. By July, the OWID graphics clearly indicated a loss of correlation and causality between the two factors, cases and deaths. This problem continued through the end of the year 2020, and now into 2021. OWID's data came from the CDC through November 30, and afterwards from Johns Hopkins University (JHU). A separate Supplemental Information PDF discusses these differing data sources.[14]

Figure 1 below shows the actual OWID graphic of *daily confirmed cases and deaths* placed together upon the same ordinate or vertical scale of numbers. The top jagged line (red on the inside front cover version) soaring upwards is the daily *cases*, while the nearly flat, horizontal black-grey line at the bottom is the daily *deaths*. As one can readily see, the plotted curve of PCR/Antigen confirmed cases is *not congruent* with the daily confirmed deaths, directly indicating they *are not, and cannot be causally linked*. The only way the confirmed case and death data might be made to appear congruent is by presenting the same data on a logarithmic scale, which boosts up smaller numbers and suppresses larger numbers. Or, the case and death data might be separated into two different graphs with the death data being exaggerated in height by several orders of magnitude. Such exaggerations misrepresent the death data as being nearly identical to the case data, when in fact they are not.

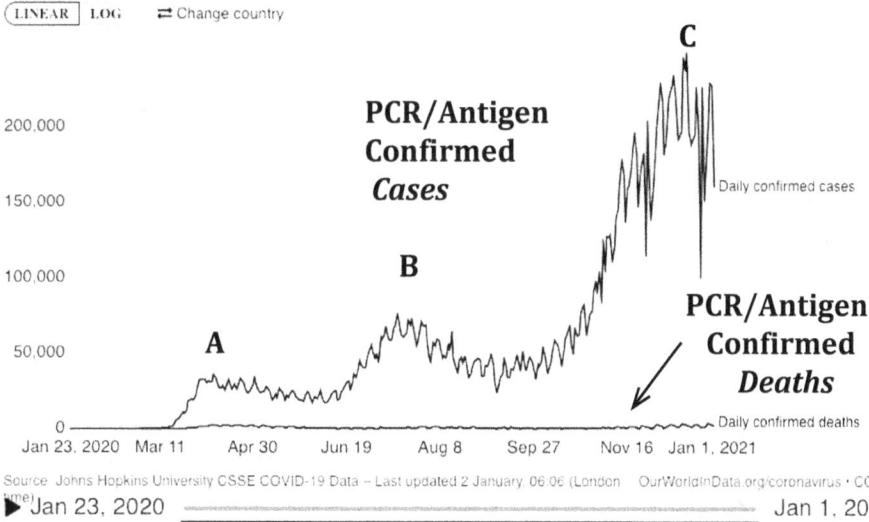

Daily confirmed COVID-19 cases and deaths, United States

The confirmed counts shown here are lower than the total counts. The main reason for this is limited testing and challenges in the attribution of the cause of death.

LINEAR LOG   ⇄ Change country

PCR/Antigen Confirmed *Cases*

PCR/Antigen Confirmed *Deaths*

A   B   C

Daily confirmed cases
Daily confirmed deaths

200,000
150,000
100,000
50,000
0

Jan 23, 2020   Mar 11   Apr 30   Jun 19   Aug 8   Sep 27   Nov 16   Jan 1, 2021

Source: Johns Hopkins University CSSE COVID-19 Data – Last updated 2 January, 06:06 (London time)   OurWorldInData.org/coronavirus • CC BY

Jan 23, 2020   Jan 1, 2021

Figure 1: Daily Covid-19 PCR/Antigen Lab-Confirmed Cases & Deaths, USA only, From early March 2020 to Jan, 1, 2021. Our World in Data website.[15]

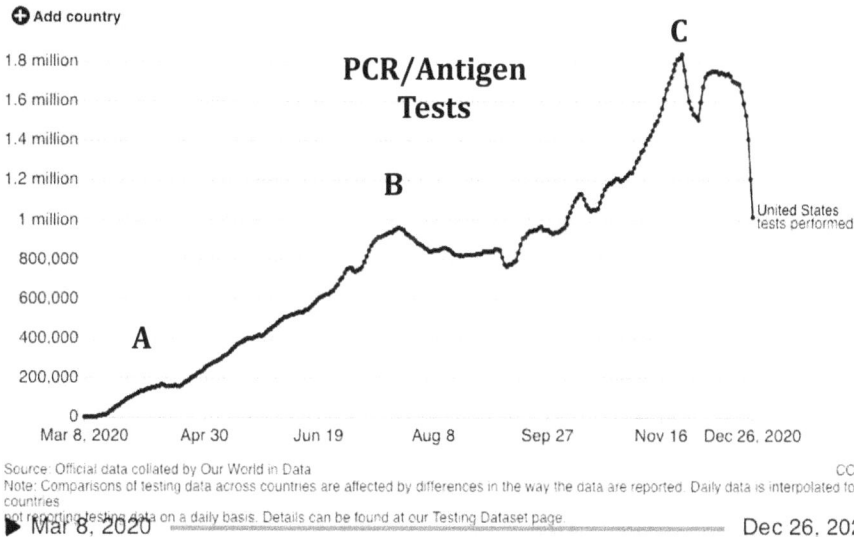

Daily COVID-19 tests

The figures are given as a rolling 7-day average.

⊕ Add country

PCR/Antigen Tests

A   B   C

United States tests performed

1.8 million
1.6 million
1.4 million
1.2 million
1 million
800,000
600,000
400,000
200,000
0

Mar 8, 2020   Apr 30   Jun 19   Aug 8   Sep 27   Nov 16   Dec 26, 2020

Source: Official data collated by Our World in Data   CC BY
Note: Comparisons of testing data across countries are affected by differences in the way the data are reported. Daily data is interpolated for countries not reporting testing data on a daily basis. Details can be found at our Testing Dataset page.

Mar 8, 2020   Dec 26, 2020

Figure 2: Daily Covid-19 PCR/Antigen Tests Administered, USA only, March 8 to Dec. 26, 2020, with 7-day averaging. Our World in Data website.[16]

17

Figure 1 clarifies the actual situation, and sets the record straight:

1. Daily Covid-19 PCR/Antigen confirmed *cases* were firstly recorded in early March, increasing over the months to dramatic numbers approaching 250,000 lab-confirmed cases per day. Three major peaks are observed in those cases: "Point A" in early to mid-April, "Point B" over the month of July, and "Point C" a third peak in confirmed cases starting in October and continuing to increase until late December and into January 2021. Lab-confirmed cases surged upwards to above 100,000 per day on Nov. 3rd, and to nearly 250,000 per day in mid-December.

2. By contrast, *the numbers of daily lab-confirmed deaths on Figure 1 have not followed such a dramatic pattern.* Out of the current US population of around 330 million, the total all-cause deaths over 2019 were ~2.85 million or ~7800 persons per day. In 2020, during the Covid crisis, the total all-cause deaths did increase, to ~3.17 million, or ~8700 persons per day. We must ask, how many of these people died in 2020 from Covid-19 versus natural causes including other diseases and conditions (their comorbidities), plus suicides or accidents? That is a primary point of discussion in this book. (See Table H on page 53 for annual all-cause death data going back 10 years.)

3. Overall *there is no significant correlation observed between the strongly surging daily confirmed cases with the relatively steady and dramatically lower numbers of daily confirmed deaths.* This is centrally important, as it reveals an inconvenient truth, that *"PCR/Antigen confirmed cases" do not indicate or predict who gets sick or remains healthy, much less who lives or who dies.* Instead, as detailed below, the variations in death numbers for the USA as a whole reveal a *seasonal pattern*, of increasing deaths in late winter of early 2020 when the Covid-19 crisis began, declining thereafter as the USA weather warmed up. A slight lesser rise in Covid-19 deaths occurred in mid-summer, as an expression of lung-irritating, hot-humid and dusty/pollen conditions afflicting susceptible people. In particular, *the dramatic increase in confirmed cases peaking in December (Point C)* shows *no corresponding dramatic increase in daily confirmed deaths.*

If the daily confirmed cases truly reflected the spread of a living airborne viral agent able to cause death in patients, then there would be a predictable and steadily increasing number of daily deaths, recording the spread of such a contagious deadly virus into the population as an increasing phenomenon. Absolute numbers of deaths would then more closely match the soaring curve of daily confirmed cases with a slight lag period. However, that is not what the Figure 1 graph reveals.

Additional answers can be found in Figure 2, presenting a graphic of daily Covid-19 *test* numbers. Figure 2 reveals a generally constant and steady increase in confirmed 7-day averaged Covid-19 PCR/Antigen *laboratory tests*, starting in early March 2020 and continuing until the end of the year. While the correlation between the curves of *test and case* numbers in these first two figures is strong, *the correlation between the curves of both test and case numbers to those of confirmed deaths is weak, nearly absent as can clearly be seen.*

4. The test-number curve of Figure 2 is in close agreement with the case numbers of Figure 1, in very specific ways. They both show a subtle bulge or increase in the numbers of tests over late March into mid April (Point A), with another slight rise from late June through July (Point B). There also is a dramatic increase in the PCR/Antigen *test and case* numbers starting in mid-October, which together reach a maximum in December (Point C).

5. The actual number of Covid-19 PCR/Antigen tests increased to a million per day in early October, reaching 1.8 million daily tests in late November, without any clear correlation to the daily deaths. The most obvious and real correlation in the Figure 1 and 2 graphs is that between the *daily PCR/Antigen laboratory tests* and *daily confirmed cases.* However, *neither of those two variables show an agreement with daily confirmed deaths, which remain at a relatively low number throughout the "pandemic".* Arguably, if a real pandemic was occurring, the lab tests would accurately predict who got sick and who remained healthy, and who lived or died, in which case, laboratory confirmed cases and death numbers would more closely correlate. *They do not.*

6. These data, when graphed, reveal a basic problem in claimed causality. At the graphical peaks in late December, at Point C, a record of around 1.8 million tests were made, detecting around 250,000 positive test reactions or cases. That is about a 14% *positive case detection rate, or about 1 person in 7.* At the same approximate time, around 3000 daily deaths were attributed to Covid-19. That works out to be one-sixteenth of one percent of *tests* (0.17%) or 1.7 per 1000 people tested. This second number is most important. Precise figures from different 15-day periods of 2020 are given below in Table A. The low probability of dying from Covid-19, viewed by such percentages, was not sufficient reason for the panic, hysteria, and loss of constitutional liberties from government-demanded masking, lockdowns and economic destruction. The following sections provide additional critical evidence on these points.

The Death/Case and Death/Test Ratios
Do Not Support a Claimed "Pandemic"

The ratio of daily laboratory-confirmed Covid-19 deaths to the daily lab-confirmed Covid-19 cases (the *death/case ratio)*, and the Covid-19 deaths versus PCR tests administered (the *death/test ratio)*, further support the criticism of *no correlation or causality*, as revealed in a separate analysis of selected 15-day periods within the Figure 1 data. Table A below presents these data in numerical form.

Table A CDC raw data (downloaded from the OWID citation for Figure 1) reveal an initial possible infectious or hysteria-driven medical and social panic, for a short-lived epoch of correlation lasting from late March (when very few were "tested"), into April (Point A) and declining in May of 2020. This is when the mainstream media was filled with fears of an escaped bat-virus from a bio-weapons lab, with all the alarming videos of crowded Chinese hospital hallways, or having dropped dead in the streets. China locked down severely, and the world "held its breath",

Table A. Death/Case & Death/Test Ratios, for 15-day periods ending on the given dates, for 2020. Raw data downloaded from Figure 1 OWID link, above.[15]						
Date 2020			Death/Case Ratio	Death/Test Ratio	D/C %	D/T %
10-Apr		1	0.051	0.01017	5.1	1.017
30-Apr	Point A	2	0.074	0.01068	7.4	1.068
25-May		3	0.057	0.00322	5.7	0.322
17-Jun		4	0.034	0.00139	3.4	0.139
10-Jul	Point B	5	0.012	0.00084	1.2	0.084
30-Jul	Point B	6	0.015	0.00106	1.5	0.106
22-Aug		7	0.021	0.00117	2.1	0.117
15-Sep		8	0.021	0.00097	2.1	0.097
4-Oct		9	0.016	0.00073	1.6	0.073
24-Oct		10	0.013	0.00069	1.3	0.069
10-Nov		11	0.009	0.00076	0.9	0.076
28-Nov		12	0.009	0.00081	0.9	0.081
15-Dec	Point C	13	0.012	0.00141	1.2	0.141
31-Dec	Point C	14	0.013	0.00160	1.3	0.160
Av. Full Year 2020:			0.0255	0.00254	2.55	0.2535
Av. July-Dec. 2020:			0.0159	0.00104	1.59	0.1039

rushing in a panic to "do something" – even though many or most of those frightening videos spread globally by major media had no independent corroboration as to their true content. One could not tell if collapsed people were drunk, victims of assault, or just plain propaganda from the Chinese Communist Party, as a calculated prelude to the WHO and CDC adoption of similar lockdown propaganda globally. PCR testing during that period was mostly confined to hospitals with already sick and suffering people having multiple symptoms congruent with the claimed SARS-CoV-2. Certainly it was SARS – Severe Acute Respiratory Syndrome – a clinical diagnosis that has been around since 2002. But, what was causing this new outbreak of SARS? A big part of it appeared to be mass panic and hysteria, driven by alarmist media reports.

The *death/case* ratios attributed to SARS-CoV-19 for those early 15-day periods of 2020 were high, peaking at 7.4% in late April, while *death/test* ratios for that same Point A were at 1%, relatively low given the fewer test numbers being made on mostly sick people. By July at Point B, as larger numbers of asymptomatic people were being tested, the death/case ratios declined to 1.2% and 1.5% with fractional death/test ratios down to 0.08% (or 8 deaths in 10,000) and 0.11% (or 11 in 10,000). The confirmed death/case and death/test ratios remained relatively low towards the year's end, at Point C, when the average December daily death/case ratios were at 1.2% and 1.3%, while the death/test ratios were about one-tenth of that, at 0.14% and 0.16%.

The average of these death/case ratios for all the above periods of 2020 works out to be 2.55%, while the more meaningful death/test ratios average at one-tenth of that figure, at 0.25%. If we exclude the early peak of 2020, and look only at the data for the period of July through December, both ratios dropped dramatically to 1.5% and 0.10% respectively.

We can add one more statistic to this analysis. With approximately 300,000 deaths, supposedly from Covid-19 disease over 2020, and a population of around 330 million, the Covid-19 *Death/Population ratio* works out to be 0.00091 (0.09%), or 9 chances in 10,000 that a person would die of claimed Covid-19 in 2020.

Again, these are not the kind of death statistics one expects during an expanding and raging infectious pandemic. In such a case, the death/case ratios would have blossomed to around 7% but continued to expand and grow over many months before receding, as the claimed infectious Covid-19 virus spread into the entire population. That never happened. The USA never experienced such crowded hospitals with people dropping dead in the street. Nobody was burying their neighbors either, no trucks slowly moving through the streets calling to "bring out your dead", as during the Medieval plagues. Nevertheless, major media and government "experts" fanned the flames of hysteria as if there was such a situation.

How else to interpret these data trends except to say the "confirmed cases" being detected by laboratory testing have *No Correlation* to the numbers or percentages of people dying. Meanwhile, the number of laboratory tests show a good or excellent correlation to the number of "confirmed cases".

These raw-data graphs indicate the PCR/Antigen tests are reacting to something in the body fluids of mostly healthy asymptomatic test subjects, but not to a living and infectious deadly virus. (Serious problems in the PCR tests are detailed in a subsequent section, starting on page 36.)

Most likely, the highly inaccurate PCR tests were and are reacting to DNA/RNA fragments and micro-cellular debris from multiple other non-infectious and dead corona virus material, plus the antibodies and suppressed antigens associated with similar exposures. Those similar exposures could include such things as colds, influenza, pneumonia, non-Covid-19 SARS and COPD antigens. This also includes dormant or dead corona virus material which has over years stimulated healthy immune system reactions within the larger population, even as at-risk elderly succumbed to such influences.

Certainly this also indicates that PCR/Antigen tests have little or no clear predictive value in determining health, sickness or death, but are largely detecting healthy biochemistry and emerging immunity from prior exposures to one or another non-lethal DNA or RNA material. More detail is presented on that issue below. The large numbers of "positive" laboratory tests are therefore primarily indicative of Herd Immunity Only, probably achieved no later than mid-year 2020. Widespread testing results as "confirmed cases" do not and never did signal any kind of persisting or resurgent deadly viral pandemic, and ought not to be misrepresented as such.

Figures 3 and 4 further confirm this interpretation of no infectious viral pandemic. They show the same graphs as in Figures 1 and 2, of daily PCR-confirmed cases, deaths and tests over 2020, but with regression lines drawn in, showing the general trend of data for all three variables.

This direct visual presentation of the data reveals a central, primary fact: The more PCR/Antigen tests being performed, the more asymptomatic "cases" are being identified, but with very few sick people and with no living or infectious virus. Such asymptomatic people are also at no risk of infecting other people. They pose no risk to public health

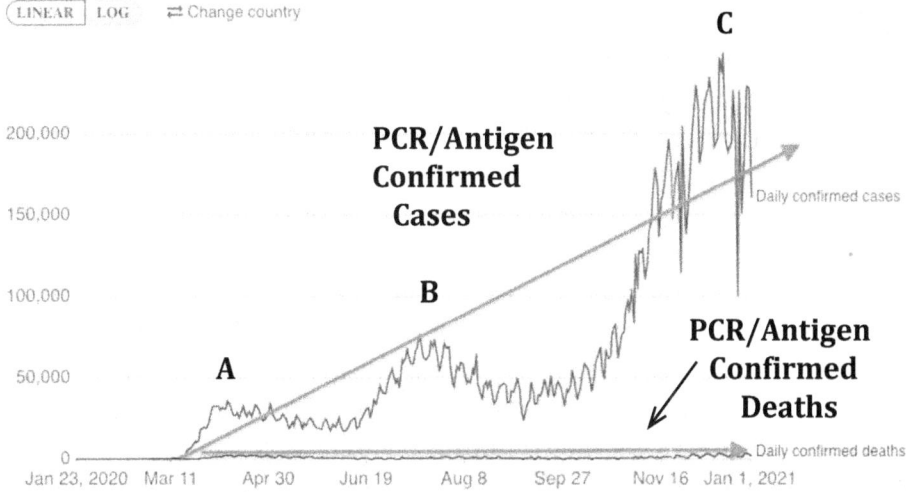

Daily confirmed COVID-19 cases and deaths, United States

The confirmed counts shown here are lower than the total counts. The main reason for this is limited testing and challenges in the attribution of the cause of death.

LINEAR LOG   ⇄ Change country

C

PCR/Antigen Confirmed Cases

B

A

PCR/Antigen Confirmed Deaths

Daily confirmed cases

Daily confirmed deaths

200,000
150,000
100,000
50,000
0

Jan 23, 2020 Mar 11   Apr 30   Jun 19   Aug 8   Sep 27   Nov 16 Jan 1, 2021

Source: Johns Hopkins University CSSE COVID-19 Data – Last updated 2 January, 06:06 (London time)   OurWorldInData.org/coronavirus • CC BY

Jan 23, 2020   Jan 1, 2021

Figure 3 (above): Daily PCR/Antigen Covid-19 Cases & Deaths[15]
(See the inside front cover for a color version)
Figure 4 (below): Daily Covid-19 PCR/Antigen Tests[16]
Same as Figures 1 and 2, but with regression lines added.

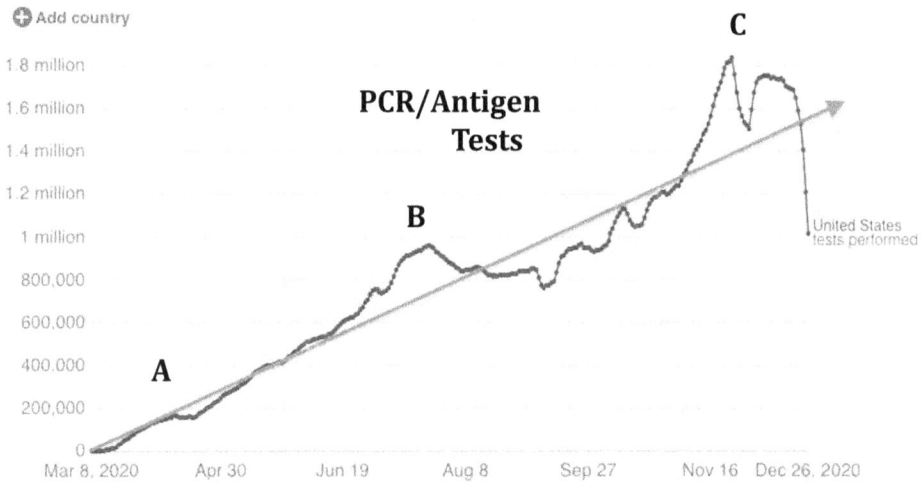

Daily COVID-19 tests

The figures are given as a rolling 7-day average.

⊕ Add country

C

PCR/Antigen Tests

B

A

United States tests performed

1.8 million
1.6 million
1.4 million
1.2 million
1 million
800,000
600,000
400,000
200,000
0

Mar 8, 2020   Apr 30   Jun 19   Aug 8   Sep 27   Nov 16 Dec 26, 2020

Source: Official data collated by Our World in Data   CC BY
Note: Comparisons of testing data across countries are affected by differences in the way the data are reported. Daily data is interpolated for countries not reporting testing data on a daily basis. Details can be found at our Testing Dataset page.

Mar 8, 2020   Dec 26, 2020

23

and identify a higher level of herd immunity within our populations than anticipated. If the Covid-19 laboratory test kits were truly accurate in detecting "confirmed cases" – reflecting a living airborne infectious virus whereby those "cases" would succumb to illness and could infect other people by aerosol exhalations, sneezing, or direct touch-contact – the confirmed deaths would have accordingly exploded to very high numbers over several months of its spread, and would today be strongly correlated to both PCR/Antigen tests and cases, and with a similar pattern in their incidence graphs. But they have not, except as misreported by medical, media and political hysterics.

Let's compare the Covid-19 death statistics to similar ones for other major causes. According to the *injuryfacts* website,[17] summarized in Table B below, the odds of dying from different causes in the USA for 2019 are set in relation to the 2020 odds of dying from Covid-19. Table B indicates "Covid-19" claimed a number of deaths somewhere between motorcycle accidents and drowning. And while similar figures for 2020 would vary to some extent, the relative odds would be approximately the same as given for 2019. And whereas those and many other causes

Table B: Lifetime odds of death for selected causes, 2019 USA[17]	
Cause of Death	Odds of Dying
Heart disease	1 in 6
Cancer	1 in 7
All preventable causes	1 in 24
Chronic lower respir. disease	1 in 27
Suicide	1 in 88
Opioid overdose	1 in 92
Fall	1 in 106
Motor-vehicle crash	1 in 107
Gun assault	1 in 289
Pedestrian incident	1 in 543
Motorcyclist	1 in 899
Covid-19 (for 2020)	**1 in 1111** (9 in 10,000)
Drowning	1 in 1128
Fire or smoke	1 in 1547
Choking on food	1 in 2535
Bicyclist	1 in 3825
Sunstroke	1 in 8248
Accidental gun discharge	1 in 8571

in this list would afflict younger people in higher percentages, Covid-19 overwhelmingly is associated with deaths among the elderly, over 80% of whom were 65 years and older, already entering the "end of life" period with multiple comorbidities. That also, as I will detail, raises serious questions about basic causality of Covid-19 disease.

Covid-19 Seasonality Does Not Support a Claimed "Pandemic"

The seasonality of Covid-19 data also supports similar conclusions, that Covid-19 diagnoses (by clinical observations or by laboratory tests) are based upon false premises, and are primarily the consequences of re-classifications of other better-known diseases and conditions that are seasonal, notably influenza, pneumonia and other pulmonary disorders, which naturally increase during wintertime. Northern and Southern Hemisphere nations also reveal a general wintertime pattern in Covid-19 data, but at opposite times of year, as shown in Figures 5 and 6. These Figures were taken directly from the OWID interactive website, and reveal a component to Covid-19 deaths which is mostly denied or ignored by the CDC, WHO, NIH, FDA and the medical community. Today it is all too obvious. Covid-19 wintertime seasonality is a confirmed fact.

Figure 5 presents a 2020 Covid-19 daily death data graph for Germany, Italy, France, Spain, Canada, Sweden, Greece and Japan, all of whom show the conventional Northern Hemisphere winter pattern. Figure 6 presents similar data for South Africa, Argentina, Chile and Australia, the most southerly Southern Hemisphere nations with significant Covid-19 deaths. New Zealand also shows a winter pattern similar to Australia, but with numbers so low they hardly show up on the graphic. Both figures reveal a clear wintertime climate pattern. Nevertheless, Covid-19 seasonality is still being hushed up by all the institutional experts, claiming everyone should just ignore the "strange ideas" as revealed in the two graphs.

As early as 28 July 2020, as "positive" lab tests began to increase, WHO released a statement through Reuters:

> **WHO says COVID-19 pandemic is 'one big wave', not seasonal**
> GENEVA (Reuters) – A World Health Organization official on Tuesday described the COVID-19 pandemic as "one big wave" and warned against complacency in the northern hemisphere summer since the infection does not share influenza's tendency to follow

Daily confirmed COVID-19 deaths, rolling 7-day average

Limited testing and challenges in the attribution of the cause of death means that the number of confirmed deaths may not be an accurate count of the true number of deaths from COVID-19.

Our World in Data

⊕ Add country

WINTER

WINTER

SUMMER

Germany
Italy
France
Spain
Canada
Sweden
Greece
Japan

800
600
400
200
0
-200

Feb 15, 2020   Apr 30   Jun 19   Aug 8   Sep 27   Nov 16   Jan 2, 2021

Source: Johns Hopkins University CSSE COVID-19 Data – Last updated 3 January, 08:00 (London time)
Note: The rolling average is the average across seven days – the confirmed deaths on the particular date, and the previous six days. For example, the value for 27th March is the average over the 21st to 27th March.

CC BY

▶ Feb 15, 2020 ◯━━━━━━━━━━━━━━━━━━━━━━━━━━◯ Jan 2, 2021

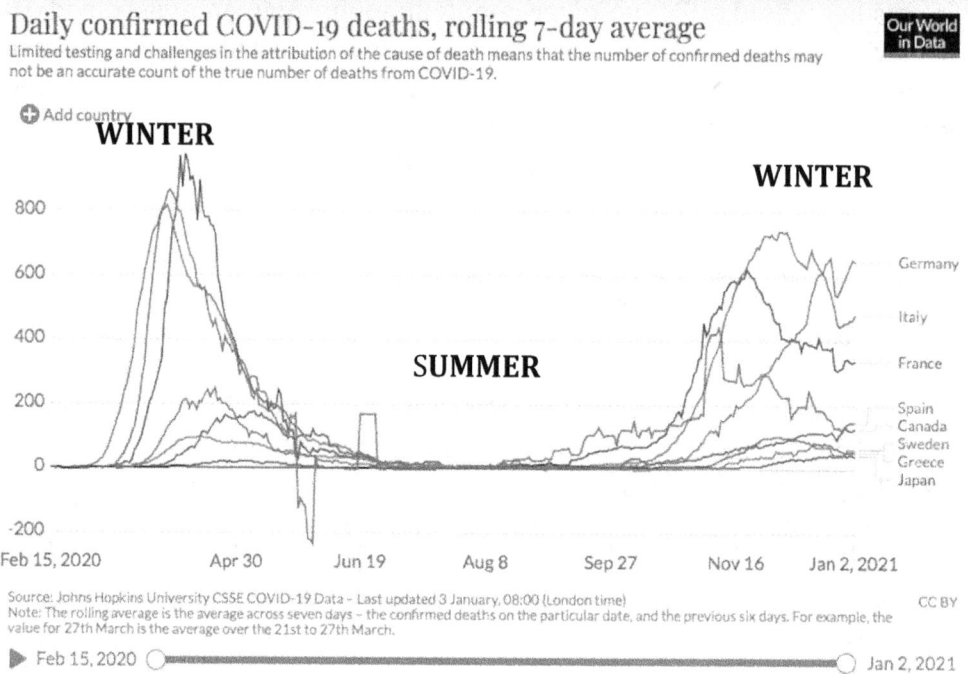

Figure 5: Covid-19 Daily Deaths, Northern Hemisphere Nations[20]
Above   (See the inside front cover for a color version)
Figure 6: Covid-19 Daily Deaths, Southern Hemisphere Nations[21]
Below

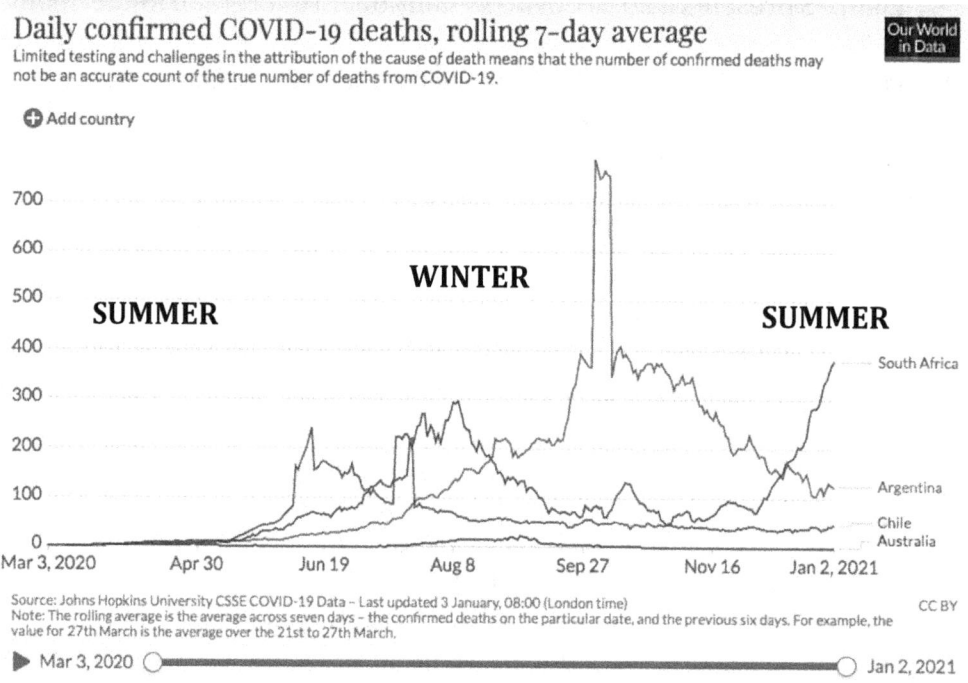

Daily confirmed COVID-19 deaths, rolling 7-day average

Limited testing and challenges in the attribution of the cause of death means that the number of confirmed deaths may not be an accurate count of the true number of deaths from COVID-19.

Our World in Data

⊕ Add country

WINTER

SUMMER

SUMMER

South Africa

Argentina
Chile
Australia

700
600
500
400
300
200
100
0

Mar 3, 2020   Apr 30   Jun 19   Aug 8   Sep 27   Nov 16   Jan 2, 2021

Source: Johns Hopkins University CSSE COVID-19 Data – Last updated 3 January, 08:00 (London time)
Note: The rolling average is the average across seven days – the confirmed deaths on the particular date, and the previous six days. For example, the value for 27th March is the average over the 21st to 27th March.

CC BY

▶ Mar 3, 2020 ◯━━━━━━━━━━━━━━━━━━━━━━━━━━◯ Jan 2, 2021

seasons. ... Pointing to high case numbers at the height of the U.S. summer, she [Margaret Harris at WHO Geneva] urged vigilance in applying measures and warned against mass gatherings. "People are still thinking about seasons. What we all need to get our heads around is this is a new virus and...this one is behaving differently," she said. "Summer is a problem. This virus likes all weather."[18]

Fortunately, the observed increase in positive test outcomes at that time was not reflected in any dramatic increase in deaths. Covid-19 deaths never came in "one big wave", but certainly the 2020 ever-increasing Covid-19 testing did.

Looking at the two figures, who are we supposed to believe – Ms. Harris of WHO? Or our "lyin' eyes"?

Here's a mid-October 2020 denial of Covid (SARS? influenza? pneumonia?) seasonality from WebMD.com.

"October 15, 2020 -- Respiratory viruses tend to be seasonal, including the two most common flu viruses, but the coronavirus that causes COVID-19 seems to be a year-round nuisance..."[19]

"Nuisance"!? "Seems to be"? Certainly it is a "year-round" problem if we look at the whole-Earth average. But individual nations and regions show different peaks of claimed Covid-19 at different times of year, based upon climatology. The issue of seasonality is a sensitive one, because by standard diagnoses, Covid-19 does indeed afflict populations quite similar to "common flu viruses", primarily, though not exclusively, during the cold-wet winter months. Covid-19 is also not easily distinguished by symptoms alone from either viral influenza or bacterial pneumonia. This issue of seasonality thereby undermines the claims of Covid-19 being caused by a new and deadly viral agent. This is well-known to epidemiologists, or should be. Today they have mostly lost their voices.

Overlap & Possible Dual- or Re-Classification
of 2020's Influenza, Pneumonia, and Other Diseases
Into the Covid-19 Category

If one has knowledge of the many basic errors in scientific or medical proofs and logic over the centuries, it is not surprising that the WHO, CDC and most other "experts" have chronically mistaken other well-known diseases and disorders as "Covid-19". Primary among these is the case of influenza. Every year, a large proportion of the elderly die of influenza, pneumonia, or other respiratory diseases. Some CDC reports appear to re-classify deaths from those long-known maladies into the Covid-19 category, or they receive a dual-classification of a single death which, alarmingly, might be counted in both categories.

Pneumonia and influenza combined claimed from 3.34% of the USA deaths in 1999 to 2.47% in 2016, on a slow declining slope, reducing them by 0.87% over that long period of 18 years, or a reduction of about 0.05% per year.[22]

Assuming that trend would continue, and extrapolating those data, the 2020 death rate from pneumonia and influenza combined would have claimed around 2.3% of USA deaths. With the total all-cause deaths at just around 3 million in 2020, that would be around 69,000 deaths. However, the same source for these pneumonia/influenza data, cited above, also has a segregated classification of "Lower Respiratory Disease" which constituted around 7% of USA deaths averaged over the 1999 to 2016 period. Extrapolating a declining trend and assuming a similar one-quarter annual reduction as given above (2.47% divided by 3.34%), the 7% average would reduce to around 5.25% of USA deaths, or 157,500 of the 3 million all cause deaths. These numbers are approximate, of course, but show the irregularities in the CDC data that, by slight changes in their categories, pneumonia, influenza and lower respiratory diseases could be either 69,000 or 157,000, or somewhere in between.

These figures add to the potential numbers of deeper-lung diseases and disorders that could easily be misdiagnosed as Covid-19, and which due to their similarities also may react positively on PCR/Antigen tests. It is admitted by physicians that diagnoses of Covid-19 are difficult to distinguish from other well-known major lung disorders. The symptoms overlap to a considerable degree, as stated on the following University of California at San Francisco Covid-19 website:

Is it possible to tell the difference between flu symptoms and COVID-19 symptoms?

"I think it's tough because both the flu and COVID-19 can have a variety of overlapping symptoms... fever, chills and body aches, upper respiratory symptoms like runny nose and sore throat, lower respiratory symptoms like cough and pneumonia, and some gastrointestinal symptoms like nausea, vomiting and diarrhea. While you could say certain symptoms are slightly more associated with one virus than the other, there's enough overlap that there's uncertainty... we wouldn't use the presence or absence of those symptoms to rule in or out either illness." [Jahan Fahimi]

"The typical symptoms of flu are relatively consistent – fever, cough and muscle aches. These are also common in COVID-19, but it's become clear as the pandemic has progressed that COVID-19 symptoms vary more wildly than those of the flu – from no symptoms at all in some 45 percent of cases to deadly pneumonia and myriad cardiovascular and neurological issues..." [Chin-Hong][23]

It is also noteworthy that, in late January 2020, the CDC was observing a dramatic increase in influenza, which had "risen for 2 consecutive weeks" and "caused at least 19 million illnesses, 180,000 hospitalizations, and 10,000 deaths so far" over the 2019-2020 winter season. However, there were only eleven Covid-19 cases in the whole USA by late January, apparently as determined by clinical diagnoses. So, what happened to that surge in influenza of January 2020? Did it continue into February and March or did it decline, or just disappear, at the same time that Covid-19 cases began to rise? And if so, is this yet another indication of Covid-19 misdiagnoses, either by clinical or PCR/Antigen confusions with influenza or other respiratory illness?[24]

An evaluation of influenza-like hospital visits for 2020 as compared to prior years is revealing, as seen in the Figures 7 and 8, page 31, taken from the CDC "Flu-View" website for week 13, April 6th, 2021. The weekly rates of hospital visits for influenza-like illness over winter 2020-2021 were between 1% to 1.5%, very low by comparison to prior years, which ranged from around 4% to 8% for the maximum months.[25] From those graphics, and other evidence, we must ask, where did the vanishing influenza go, if not by re-definition into Covid-19? And how many other diseases and disorders were also magically transformed into Covid-19?

I have yet to read any convincing conventional Covid-19 explanation for this *Mystery of the Incredible Vanishing Influenza*, as shown in Figure 7 below. Over the wintertime of 2020-2021, typically expected but very vague "influenza-associated" or "influenza-like" cases declined dramatically, even as "Covid-19 cases" soared. Consider the following January 1st 2021 interview with epidemiologist Knut Wittkowski, former head of Biostatistics, Epidemiology and Research Design at Rockefeller University:

> "Influenza has been renamed COVID in large part ...There may be quite a number of influenza cases included in the 'presumed COVID' category of people who have COVID symptoms which Influenza symptoms can be mistaken for, but are not tested for SARS RNA ... [Those patients] also may have some SARS RNA sitting in their nose while being infected with Influenza, in which case the influenza would be 'confirmed' to be COVID." [26]

CDC websites also reveal a common lumping of pneumonia and influenza with Covid-19, into the same categories. For example, on a "Flu-View" website presenting the incidence of pneumonia and influenza by week, produced by the National Center for Health Statistics Mortality Surveillance, they speak about the "Percent P&I" (pneumonia and influenza) in text and on the ordinate (vertical) scale of a dominant graphic.[27] However, another website from the CDC presenting similar text and nearly identical graphics has reclassified "P&I" into "Percent due to PIC", lumping together pneumonia, influenza and Covid-19. The ordinate or vertical scale is rebranded also, from the above earlier "% of All Deaths Due to P&I" to "% of All Deaths Due to PIC". Other irregularities are present.[28]

These overlaps and mixing of influenza, pneumonia and Covid-19 are quite apparent on the CDC's weekly reports, as seen in the Figure 8 banner identifying variant group definitions. While the banner reveals all deaths involving Covid-19 (defined by code U07.1), it also lists several categories that mix Covid-19 with influenza and/or pneumonia, either individually or together. However, the CDC did not show the isolated figures for influenza, pneumonia or Covid-19 independently, *without mixing them up*, which would be the proper method for an authentic scientific review of what are claimed to be different maladies, with different causes.

This Figure 8 banner was removed from the above CDC website in

Influenza–Associated Hospitalizations:

Between October 1, 2020, and April 3, 2021, FluSurv-NET sites in 14 states reported 215 laboratory confirmed influenza hospitalizations for an overall cumulative hospitalization rate of 0.7 per 100,000 population. This is much lower than average for this point in the season and lower than rates for any season since routine data collection began in 2005, including the low severity 2011-12 season. The current rate is one-eighth the rate at this time during the 2011-12 season. Hospitalization rates stratified by age will be presented if case counts increase to a level that produces stable rates by age.

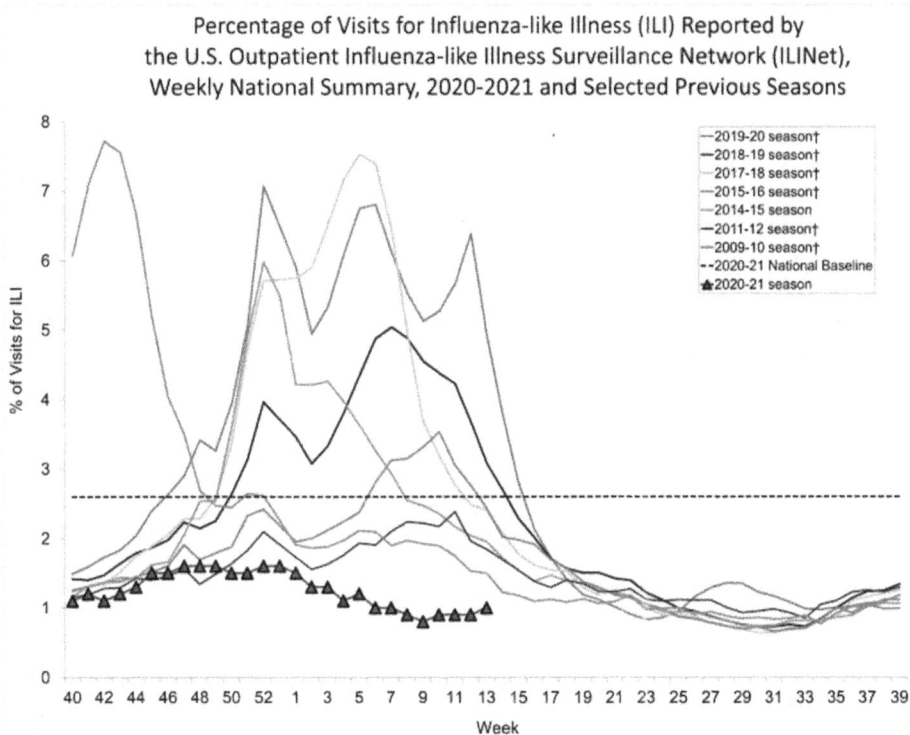

Percentage of Visits for Influenza-like Illness (ILI) Reported by the U.S. Outpatient Influenza-like Illness Surveillance Network (ILINet), Weekly National Summary, 2020-2021 and Selected Previous Seasons

Figure 7: Percentages of outpatient "influenza-like" treatments over the 2020-2021 winter season, compared to prior winter seasons back to 2009. The dark triangles are for 2020-2021.[27] (See the inside rear cover for a color version of this graphic.)

Sex	Age group	All Deaths involving COVID-19 (U07.1)[1]	Deaths from All Causes	Deaths involving Pneumonia, with or without COVID-19, excluding Influenza deaths (J12.0–J18.9)[2]	Deaths involving COVID-19 and Pneumonia, excluding Influenza (U07.1 and J12.0–J18.9)[2]	All Deaths involving Influenza, with or without COVID-19 or Pneumonia (J09–J11)[3]	Deaths involving Pneumonia, Influenza, or COVID-19 (U07.1 or J09–J18.9)[4]	Population[5]

Figure 8: Multiple Accountings for Influenza, Pneumonia and Covid-19 [30]

early February 2021 and replaced by a slightly different one., a little less confusing, but nevertheless revealing the mix-ups.

Under the heading "Comorbidities and Other Conditions", a "Table 3" section of the same weblink above, presented a very long list of exactly what other diseases and disorders people with a positive PCR/Antigen "confirmed case" or "confirmed death" were suffering from. Here are those categories, "contributing to deaths where Covid-19 was listed on the death certificate". [30]

Influenza and pneumonia
Chronic lower respiratory diseases
Adult respiratory distress syndrome
Respiratory failure
Respiratory arrest
Other diseases of the respiratory system
Hypertensive diseases
Ischematic (poor circulation) heart disease
Cardiac arrest
Heart Failure
Cerebrovascular diseases
Other diseases of the circulatory system
Sepsis
Malignant neoplasm
Diabetes
Obesity
Alzheimer disease
Vascular and unspecified dementia
Renal failure
Intentional or unintentional injury, poisoning and
    other adverse events
All other conditions and causes (residual)
Covid-19 (by laboratory PCR/Antigen tests, or clinical diagnoses)

That same CDC website further divided the above listing into age groups, from which even a cursory look indicated the overwhelming majorities were in age groups of 55 and older. The maximum numbers were in the two oldest categories, of 75-84 years, and 85 and older. These are people reaching the end-of-life period, suffering from multiple comorbidities, which again raises the question of just what they died of.

The pre-February 2021 CDC data did not answer the centrally important question of how many people died of a strictly Covid-19 diagnosis, as per PCR/Antigen testing, without pneumonia, influenza or other comorbidities. However, that question was cleared up in the CDC's post-February 2021 clarification of their data presentations at that same Figure 8 website.

> *"For over 5% of these deaths, Covid-19 was the only cause mentioned on the death certificates. For deaths with conditions or causes in addition to Covid-19, on average, there were 4.0 additional conditions or causes per death."* [30]

The above post-February iteration of that CDC webpage listed Covid-19 data for the entire periods of 2020 and 2021, through 11 April as of my last review. It indicated a total of 543,161 people had died of Covid-19. But only 5% or 27,158 died only of Covid-19, without any of the other average 4 different causes or comorbidities as given on the death certificates. That figure covers a period of around 13 months, from the start of March 2020 through the end of March 2021, or about 2,089 purely Covid-19 deaths per month, or about 68 deaths per day for the US in total. Or, about 1.4 deaths per day, per state, on average.

By February 2021, I estimated that most of the Covid-19 deaths must be afflicted with more than one or two comorbidities, given how two or three of those individual categories, when added together, exceeded the total Covid-19 deaths many times over. The CDC finally confirmed my suspicions, but the situation they presented with an average of 4 comorbidities per Covid-19 death is even worse than what I anticipated.

Again, *what is going on in these different presentations of the same data, if not a re-definition and shifting of pneumonia, influenza and other broad categories of significant deaths into a Covid-19 classification,* either in whole or in part? At best, it reveals diagnostic difficulties and confusion. At worst, it is *Very Bad Science, with possible implications of fraud.*

This question, of how many people died of Covid-19 only, without comorbidities, was first raised in a paper by Ealy, et al. dated to October 2020. They wrote:

> "According to the Centers for Disease Control and Prevention (CDC) on August 23, 2020, 'For 6% of the deaths, COVID-19 was the only cause mentioned. For deaths with conditions or causes in addition to COVID-19 , on average, there were 2.6 additional conditions

or causes per death.' ... For a nation tormented by restrictive public health policies mandated for healthy individuals and small businesses, this is the most important statistical revelation of this crisis. This revelation significantly impacts the published fatalities count due to COVID-19."[8]

Ealy et al. also produced a time-line of CDC methods for acquiring and reporting of epidemic deaths, revealing how in February 2020, CDC changed its method of data collection and counting (as in the _Medical Examiners' and Coroners' Handbook on Death Registration_ and the _Physician's Handbook on Medical Certification of Death_) thereby abandoning a methodology they had successfully employed nationwide since 2003. From February 2020 onward, the CDC's data reports on Covid-19 became increasingly confusing and obscure, and by Ealy, et al., "violated data quality, objectivity, utility and integrity requirements". By using the 2003 methods of computing Covid-19 fatalities, the conclusions given in the above Abstract of 6% of deaths being due only to Covid-19, without comorbidities, were founded.[8]

The full 2020 year end total USA Covid-19 deaths with comorbidities was 313,171 (see my Figure 13, p.52 and Table H, p.53). By the Ealy et al. 6% calculation that number suddenly drops to **18,790 deaths for the full year**, which works out to be 52 deaths per day, for all 50 US states. About 1 death, per state, per day. _That is very close to the determination as finally admitted by the CDC in their post-February 2021 revised data calculations of "over 5%", as I quoted above._ Whether one endorses the Ealy, et al computation, or my computation above based upon the post-February CDC data, they together present a dramatically different picture of this "pandemic" than what is given by "official sources". In a subsequent section, I developed an even better, more accurate and robust method for calculating "excess deaths" due to claimed Covid-19, using the CDC's own data, with an even lower net estimate, as given on pages 58-59.

More Errors: Electron Microscope Image Confusions?

Visual identifications of the claimed "novel" (unique) SARS-CoV-2 in the electron microscope reveal variations which, to my eye as a skilled microscopist[31] and probably to many others, suggest *different viral entities*. Electron micrograph images of claimed SARS-CoV-2 are also *not so clearly different* from other corona viruses typical of influenza, pneumonia or other respiratory diseases. Figure 9 shows two dissimilar images of claimed SARS-CoV-2 virus, as obtained from NIH/NIAID. Aside from the false-color variations added to enhance their contrasts, without clarifications, they do not appear to be the same viral entities. A caption with these images revealed the difficulty in making assessments of what is SARS-CoV-2 and what is something else:

> "... the images do not look much different from MERS-CoV (Middle East respiratory syndrome coronavirus, which emerged in 2012) or the original SARS-CoV (Severe Acute Respiratory Syndrome coronavirus, which emerged in 2002). That is not surprising: The spikes on the surface of corona viruses give this virus family its name – corona, which is Latin for "crown," and most any coronavirus will have a crown-like appearance."[32]

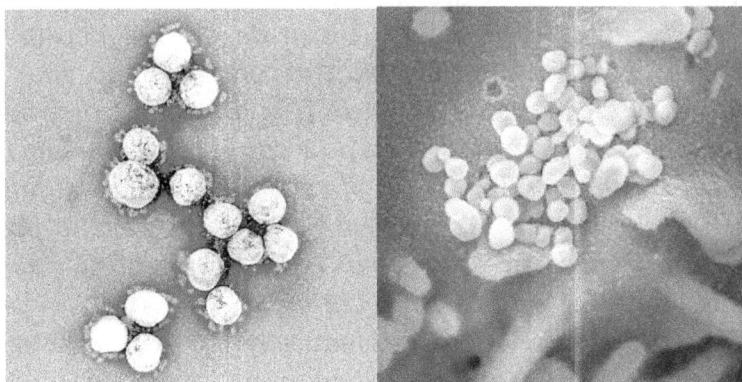

**Figure 9: Two Dissimilar Images of
Claimed SARS-CoV-2.** (NIH/NIAID)[20]

For reference, similar viral images appear on the NIAID's MERS-CoV page.[33] Another website also shows many different electron micrograph images of claimed SARS-CoV-2, only some of which appear identical to others.[34] Be your own judge.

The Fallacy of PCR/Antigen Testing "Accuracy"

The PCR, or *Polymerase Chain Reaction* testing method, is a biochemical process whereby billions of copies of a DNA/RNA molecular strand in a test sample can be replicated. The process employs a chemical solution of polymerase mixed with a person's body fluids, which are then subjected to repeated cycles of thermal heating and cooling. The polymerase reactant binds to DNA/RNA strands and replicates their biochemical patterns as the temperatures cycle up and down. By doing so, tiny and otherwise undetectable traces of DNA/RNA can be artificially replicated and magnified *a billion times over,* in quantities sufficient for study. Fluorescent dyes are also added which chemically bond to the amplified genetic material. When exposed to ultraviolet light, the intensity of fluorescence is claimed to indicate the quantity of the claimed "toxic" DNA/RNA in the sample.

Originally undertaken as a lengthy hands-on laboratory process, PCR magnification is today automated, undertaken in specialized laboratory machinery which yields a variable "quantity" of the PCR-amplified DNA/RNA. When used for clinical diagnoses, however, all kinds of serious problems arise. It does not give a "yes or no" result, as with a pregnancy test, but instead gives a relative measure, where results above a subjectively declared value are claimed to be "positive". Slightly below that is "negative". That is the theory. The primary problem is this:

If you only have such a tiny quantity of a virus in your system which requires PCR methods to magnify it a billion times over so it can be detected and identified, then how can it have any biochemical significance or effect upon your physiology in the original non-amplified tiny quantity? And doesn't that indicate, the presumed living and dangerous infectious virus is NOT replicating itself? And therefore is NOT alive, and NOT infectious?

Those questions have been systematically ignored or forbidden by "PCR Testing Kit" advocates and profit-seeking pharmaceutical companies, starting in the AIDS years when PCR tests were yielding false positives on claimed "HIV" in abundance. Even at a time when people were dying of multiple AIDS-indicator diseases (AIDS comorbidities), direct detection of HIV in their bodies was often impossible, and could only occur with PCR billion magnifications. But there are other major scientific reasons why *SARS-CoV-2 PCR testing is specifically flawed, and has no objective value for clinical diagnoses.*[35,36,37,38]

1. PCR tests cannot distinguish between a living infectious virus and a dead virus of the same or similar type. *It will yield a positive indication when detecting DNA or RNA fragments from the break-down products of a multitude of viral entities similar to the one the test is supposed to be looking for.* This is why vast numbers of asymptomatic people with zero living SARS-CoV-2 in their systems are getting false-positive results from these tests. It is also why, after taking the new breed of mRNA vaccines which inject such genetic material into a person's system, it lingers and hence shows up on subsequent PCR tests, suggesting vaccinated people are still at risk of Covid-19 disease. Or, as I believe, the post-vaccination PCR test is merely magnifying what was injected into their bodies. Whatever the reason, this was never predicted by the vaccine hysterics, who are today required to jump through hoops in order to "explain" or "explain away" what is going on in their vaccinated kennels.

2. As previously noted, SARS-CoV-2 virus is very similar in appearance and symptoms to other corona viruses as associated with respiratory disorders. How can we be certain if the PCR is detecting SARS-CoV-2, or any other corona virus? Or, if PCR is identifying living virus or remnant dead viral matter from our immune-system destruction of it? Or if it is reacting to our own antibodies to various corona viruses, to which we have become immune over many years? We cannot know. PCR does not give such answers. It is like a very low-resolution video camera that is supposed to ring an alarm bell whenever a burglar comes to your front door. But it can't distinguish between a "burglar" or you or your children, the postman, or even the neighbor's dog or cat. It reacts to all of them.

3. The outcome of a Covid-19 PCR "test" is dependent upon the number of thermal heating and cooling cycles a sample is put through, and that is determined by settings on the machine which the laboratory technician can adjust, for more or fewer thermal cycles. If this *cycle threshold* (CT) is set too high, the added cycles will replicated additional tens of millions of DNA or RNA strands in the sample, yielding higher rates of "positive" reactions. A setting of 25 cycles is considered rather low and will yield fewer or no "positive" replications. More than 30 cycles is considered scientifically bogus, with higher percentages of "positives". However, the FDA, CDC and WHO have variously recommended PCR test machinery be set at 35 to 40 cycles! Under such circumstances, one can view all "positive PCR tests" as laboratory artifacts, or "false positives".

Problems as these are why some PCR testing labs around the country have reported 100% positives for entire populations. This created a major scandal in Florida, where several labs were consistently reporting

100% Covid-19 results, alerting Governor DeSantis to their bogus nature, leading to an end of the lockdowns "Covid experts" had been advising.[39]

Kary Mullis, who invented the PCR method of DNA/RNA amplification and won a Nobel Prize in Chemistry in 1993 for doing so, did not accept the HIV theory of AIDS due to its heavy reliance upon PCR magnification to prove its existence.[40] In an endorsement for fellow scientist Peter Duesberg, he once declared "We know that to err is human, but the HIV/ AIDS hypothesis is one hell of a mistake. I say this rather strongly as a warning." Duesberg, a top virologist at UC Berkeley, was highly critical of the HIV theory of AIDS, arguing it was a harmless "passenger retrovirus",[74] while other AIDS critics considered HIV to be a non-existing creation of haphazard PCR magnifications. Significantly, *no pure culture isolation has been made of either HIV or SARS-CoV-2,* nor of other corona viruses.

Duesberg and all the AIDS critics were severely punished professionally and subjected to widespread medical-media slander and censorship. Mullis, who died in 2019, was basically excommunicated from the world of science for his public criticisms of PCR methods and the HIV theory of AIDS, even as various biotech companies, but not Mullis, raked in billions from his discovery.

Today, the same big problems and inaccurate claims that emerged during the bogus "HIV epidemic" (which was supposed to depopulate Africa by now), have come back once again under the umbrella of Covid-19. The SARS-CoV-2 theory of Covid-19 disease (or of ordinary SARS, influenza, pneumonia, and other "comorbidities" lumped together under the "Covid-19" umbrella) must be viewed in a similar manner. The conditions or diseases called SARS or influenza, etc., are very real, and can be deadly. However, SARS-CoV-2 virus theory has no unambiguous evidence of *causing* such diseases.

Most interesting on PCR is how, in early January 2021, the WHO issued an Information Notice exposing its lack of accuracy, stating:

"WHO reminds [lab workers] that disease prevalence alters the predictive value of test results; as disease prevalence decreases, the risk of false positive increases...This means that the probability that a person who has a positive result (SARS-CoV-2 detected) is truly infected with SARS-CoV-2 decreases as prevalence decreases, *irrespective of the claimed specificity.*"[41]

And in a similarly outrageous manner, in early May 2021 the CDC released a fact sheet on "COVID-19 vaccine breakthrough case investigation

– Information for public health, clinical, and reference laboratories".[42] A "breakthrough case" occurs when a person tests positive for Covid-19 *after* being vaccinated. The fact sheet directed PCR testing labs to use a *low cycle threshold (CT) of only 28 for previously vaccinated people.* This procedural change would insure fewer of the vaccinated would subsequently "test positive". However, the unstated assumption was, that the unvaccinated would continue to be tested with a CT as usual, at 35 to 40 cycles, *insuring the unvaccinated group would continue to show high levels of PCR false-positive tests.* But in fact, it is the vaccinated who seem to suffer the greater problems flowing from bogus PCR testing. Previously vaccinated people continue to "test positive" and if they die, their deaths are then blamed on "Covid-19" (rather than the vaccines). This is today a huge embarrassment for the Covid-hysterics and vaccine companies, as it reveals they have no idea what they are doing. The CDC inadvertently exposed their fraud to the public eye, in a criminal manner apparently designed to punish the unvaccinated refuseniks, and artificially inflate the numbers of "positive unvaccinated Covid-19 cases".[42]

Antigen test kits similarly rely upon biochemical factors, but more directly react to viral membrane components. They are quicker in their analysis and truly more accurate than PCR. But the medical industry considers them less reliable, with claimed "high levels of false negatives", because PCR routinely yields higher positive tests. The claimed inaccuracy of antigen testing is blamed upon invisible "hiding virus" that antigen tests cannot detect, but which PCR can detect. This reasoning is sophistry, however, as it excludes the possibility that there isn't any "hiding virus" at all, and that PCR tests are reacting to all kinds of other things. It is simply an inconvenient truth that antigen test kits show far fewer "positives" than the doctors anticipate (or wish for?). Additionally, antigens and antibodies can reside in the same host, indicating a healthy and successful immune-system termination of the toxic element. The antigen tests are therefore no better than PCR in "confirming" living infectious virus.

There are other factors that can lead to a positive Covid-19 diagnosis, testing or not. Statements made by many physicians on internet and in video interviews, including by Senator Scott Jensen of Minnesota (also a physician) have identified at least one motivation for doing so: *large sums of money are given to hospitals by Medicare and other Federal agencies when they take on a new Covid-19 patient who is placed on a ventilator, around $39,000 in total.*[43] Jensen's video statement has since been censored by YouTube, but the *USA Today* newspaper and FactCheck.org launched separate investigations of the subject, confirming his analysis.

"Hospital administrators might well want to see COVID-19 attached to a discharge summary or a death certificate. Why? Because if it's a straightforward, garden-variety pneumonia that a person is admitted to the hospital for – if they're Medicare – typically, the diagnosis-related group lump sum payment would be $5,000. But if it's COVID-19 pneumonia, then it's $13,000, and if that COVID-19 pneumonia patient ends up on a ventilator, it goes up to $39,000."[43]

Senator/Doctor Jensen has since gone on to make other sharp criticisms of conventional medicine related to Covid-19, and an internet search on his name plus "Covid-19" will pull up many articles and videos. But his initial revelations on Covid-19 financing further suggest many Covid-19 deaths are being classified twice, firstly by physicians on the real comorbidity cause of their deaths (influenza, pneumonia, lung cancer, diabetes, etc.) and later as Covid-19, by the determinations of hospital staff and administrators, or by the CDC itself.

At this point, we may pause, and consider how all the above facts have seriously undermined the theoretical Covid-19/SARS-CoV-2 paradigm. Virtually *none* of the claims of a new and unique causality, of toxicity from a claimed SARS-CoV-2 virus, can be reconciled with the critical facts presented so far. The various comorbidities are well known and documented over decades, but the claimed infectious Covid-19 disease is not. Below in the next section, I present CDC confirmed-death data in Tables H, I and J, casting further doubt upon the exclusive and singular claim of a deadly infectious viral pandemic destroying the lives of people at high numbers. The data is focused upon the USA, but by inference and extrapolation, the arguments apply globally. Many lives are lost or being destroyed, but we must ask if this is more due to severe anxiety, panic, hysteria, forced lockdowns, economic ruin and attending social chaos, than by a claimed infectious SARS-CoV-2 viral pandemic.[44]

We must look to *other reasons* for the excess deaths of 2020 and early 2021, being mis-attributed to a "Covid-19 pandemic." Those other reasons, I will show, are the product of human ignorance, error and malice, in government-medical demands for massive social changes which took a terrible toll in human isolation, misery and despair.

The Real Pandemic – Death Toll from Forced Lockdowns, Toxic Masking, Economic Ruin & *Deaths by Despair*

In spite of political, medical and media misrepresentations, there is no clear evidence that shows locking down entire societies, disrupting economies or forcing everyone under contaminated oxygen-depriving masks does anything of benefit towards mitigation against claimed Covid-19. The best review of this was presented in a now-banned YouTube video by Ivor Cummins, who also expanded upon the issue of seasonality.[45] Unfortunately, rather than stimulating debate, YouTube censored the Cummins video, as they do with anything critical of conventional Covid theory, but it has been saved elsewhere as a download.[46]

Cummins' video presented various data graphics showing how daily Covid-19 deaths were already on a clear downward trend at the time when many of the nation-wide or USA state-wide lockdowns were instituted. Cummins' argued that implementing or ending of lockdowns had no significant effect upon Covid-19 deaths, either to increase or decrease them significantly. However, within the states and nations he reviewed, all showed the above-noted trends of increased Covid-19 deaths as the weather turned damp and cold, and decreased deaths as it turned dry and warm. States which locked down most ferociously often had the most intensive spikes in death afterwards, due to the secondary health issues created by lockdowns and masking. In example, the state of Florida, whose Governor DeSantis basically ended all lockdowns and forced-masking laws in late September 2020, experienced a gradual lowering Covid-19 death rates, as shown in Figure 10 below. Covid-19 deaths did not subsequently increase.

Additionally, as seen in Figure 11, Florida (the bar at bottom) compared more favorably than strong lockdown states such as OR, MA, CA, KY, IL, MI, OH, NM and MN. Florida had lower rates of cases, hospitalization and deaths. This list is selective and incomplete, but the reader will understand the point, that critical complaints to end lockdowns and masking have significant facts to back them up, indicating there is little or no benefit to public health by lockdowns and forced masking policies. This figure was reproduced by Cummins from a NY Times web resource which has since removed (*censored!*) the comparative information.[47]

A similar situation was observed in the state of Texas, where in late April Governor Abbot ended lockdowns amid a storm of criticism that death numbers would skyrocket. Instead, they fell to very low single-digit death numbers by late May. A similar story is found in South Dakota, where Governor Noem refused to order any lockdowns. Same with Idaho, Montana and Georgia, all with minimal government edicts on lockdowns, masking or social distancing. Retail stores, restaurants, salons, barber shops, churches, gyms and outdoor recreation proceeded there as normal, and children resumed in-classroom education without fanfare or catastrophe. They did not suffer any increase in deaths because of it, their death-case ratios ranged between 1.1% and 1.7%. By contrast, in the most severely locked-down states such as New York, Pennsylvania, New Jersey, Massachusetts or New York City, death-case ratios ranged between 2.6% to 4.4%, *more than double the no-lockdown states.* The numbers on this are shown in Table C.

The averages between these two sets of states indicates a doubling of death/case ratios in the Severe Lockdown States, by comparison to the No-

Table C: Preliminary Covid-19 Death/Case Ratios in Selected Locked Versus Unlocked States[47]			
As of 5 Feb.2021	Total Covid Cases	Total Covid Deaths	Covid-19 Death/Case Ratio
NO OR MILD LOCKDOWN STATES			
Florida	1,700,000	27,456	1.6%
Georgia	909,170	14,413	1.6%
Idaho	165,058	1,760	1.1%
Montana	95,539	1,312	1.4%
South Dakota	109,132	1,804	1.7%
Texas	2,400,000	39,320	1.6%
Averages:	896,483	14,344	1.5%
SEVERE LOCKDOWN STATES			
Massachusetts	537,208	14,859	2.8%
Michigan	619,150	15,739	2.5%
New Jersey	713,324	21,886	3.1%
New York	1,400,000	44,210	3.2%
New York City	632,306	27,609	4.4%
Pennsylvania	871,435	22,422	2.6%
Averages:	795,571	24,454	3.1%
Av. Deaths in Severe Lockdown states times 25 =			611,354
Av. Deaths in No- or Mild Lockdown states times 25=			358,604
DEATH DIFFERENCE			**252,750**

or Mild Lockdown States, from 1.5% to 3.1%. Extrapolating, if we make a general assumption that the number of lockdown and no-lockdown USA states is approximately equal (25 of each) and then multiply each of the average number of deaths using these extreme cases as a guideline, a very general and preliminary calculation can be made as to how many people died in the locked-down states, above those in no-lockdown states.

*This incomplete and abbreviated analysis suggests **over 250,000 extra deaths** across the Severe Lockdown States, which might not have occurred had they adopted milder government-demanded lockdowns, or no lockdowns at all.* And by "Severe Lockdowns" I reference the spectrum of

Figure 10: Lack of Increase in Florida Deaths After End of Lockdowns[46]

New Deaths from COVID-19 per Day by States/Territories, normalized by population

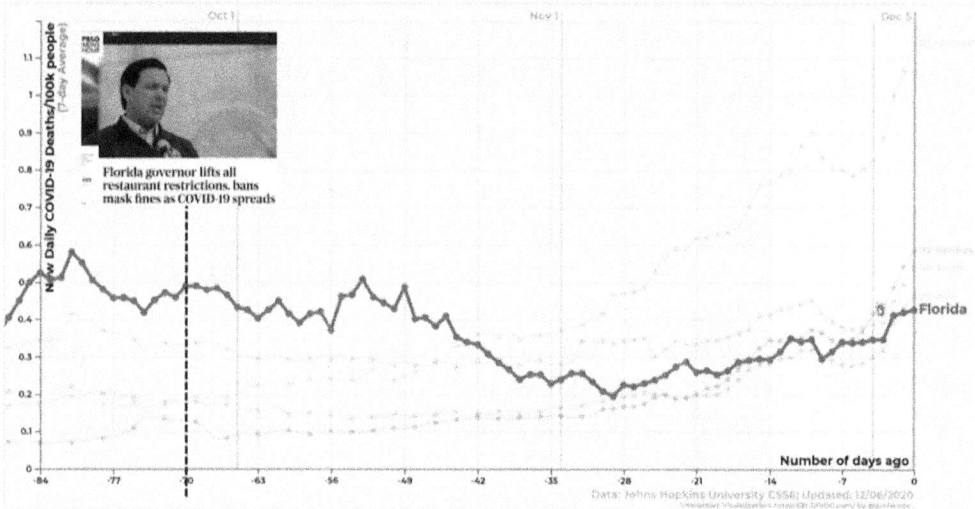

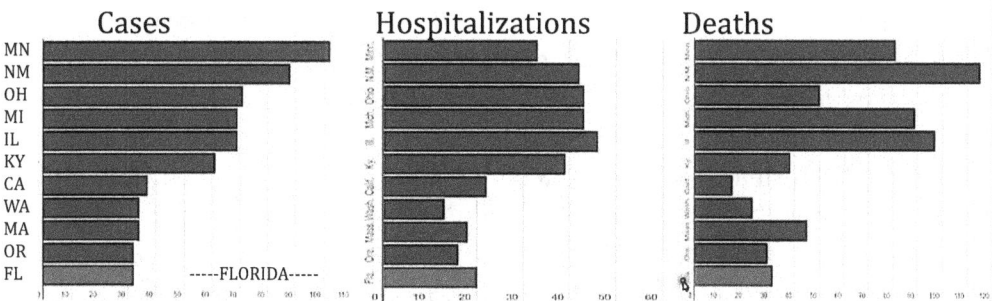

Figure 11: Selected State's Morbidity & Mortality Due to Claimed Covid-19[46] (Florida is at the chart bottom)

demands including business closures, forced masking, inhuman antisocial distancing, closure of schools, sports, concerts, public gatherings in parks or on the beach, and the subsequent severe economic destruction, bankruptcies, agony, drug overdoses, suicides, etc., that were forthcoming as society was shut down by totalitarian government edicts.

This is an incomplete analysis, but is telling on what is to be expected in a more in-depth national assessment. Some states with severe lockdowns, such as Oregon or Washington also have death/case ratios similar to the no-lockdown states. But I could not find a no-lockdown state with higher death/case ratios. This analysis adds support to the point that locking down entire states or nations in an extreme manner has no benefits, creating even worse conditions for their citizens, with *more* deaths, not fewer. *This also strongly indicates that Covid-19 is NOT an infectious disorder.*

Greater determining variables, more powerful than claimed Covid-19 disease – such as cold winter weather, the percentage of older people in a given state, and an abundance of comorbidities in older age groups being mistaken as Covid-19 by inaccurate diagnoses and flawed PCR/Antigen tests – produce these variable death numbers. Florida for example has more older folk than other states, but also milder winters. People spend a lot more time out in the Sun getting good exposure for vitamin D synthesis. A healthy diet and vitamin intake, especially C and D, are great preventives for all kinds of respiratory illness. Other states such as New York engaged in brutal measures against their older people, moving the elderly with multiple comorbidities from hospitals into nursing homes, and promoting with fanfare the use of often-deadly ventilators and denial of effective medicines. Today we know NY State was undercounting their death numbers, to boost up the sagging popularity of their Gov. Cuomo.

Whatever else may be at work, graphical confirmed case data for most states as given at the above cited NY Times website, nearly all show the wintertime seasonal pattern of incidence, as discussed above. Several webpages identify and provide links to different published studies in science or medical journals that refute benefits of lockdowns as well as exposing their deadly consequences.[14,48] Such studies indicate the most life-protective approach would demand NO lockdowns, forced masking and the like, to never start them. But that was not to happen.

In 2019 (pre-Covid-19) the WHO issued pandemic guidelines that explicitly forbade – "Not recommended in any circumstances" – the use of "Contact tracing, Quarantine of exposed individuals, Entry and exit screening, Internal travel restrictions, Border Closures".[5] This statement, reproduced below in Figure 12, was for both epidemic and pandemic circumstances. We must ask: *Why did the WHO change their recommendations less than a year before Covid-19?* And why did the world's leaders and even freedom-oriented populations so sheepishly or enthusiastically go along with the lockdown, masking and economic ruin demanded by these over-bloated government agencies?

Tables D and E, to follow, are taken from the CollateralGlobal website organized by a collection of British and American university professors and associates, working privately outside of government. They provide a summary of the horrors inflicted by forced lockdowns, masking and inhuman anti-social distancing.

Table 1. Recommendations on the use of NPIs by severity level

SEVERITY	PANDEMIC*	EPIDEMIC
Any	Hand hygiene Respiratory etiquette Face masks for symptomatic individuals Surface and object cleaning Increased ventilation Isolation of sick individuals Travel advice	Hand hygiene Respiratory etiquette Face masks for symptomatic individuals Surface and object cleaning Increased ventilation Isolation of sick individuals Travel advice
Moderate	*As above, plus* Avoiding crowding	*As above, plus* Avoiding crowding
High	*As above, plus* Face masks for public School measures and closures	*As above, plus* Face masks for public School measures and closures
Extraordinary	*As above, plus* Workplace measures and closures Internal travel restrictions	*As above, plus* Workplace measures and closures
Not recommended in any circumstances	UV light Modifying humidity Contact tracing Quarantine of exposed individuals Entry and exit screening Border closure	UV light Modifying humidity Contact tracing Quarantine of exposed individuals Entry and exit screening Internal travel restrictions Border closure

NPI: non-pharmaceutical intervention; UV: ultraviolet.

Figure 12: WHO's 2019 Recommendations for Pandemic Reduction,[5] *Abandoned in 2020!?*

Table D: Mental & Social Health[49]

Categories of Increased Collateral Damage from Covid-19 due to Hysteria, Lockdowns, Forced Masking. Reports are from peer-reviewed research in the UK unless otherwise noted

Addiction & Substance Abuse – 39% relapse of recovered addicts, 1 million affected; 34% increase in anti-anxiety meds in USA; 33% to 38% increase in alcohol consumption with increased alcohol-related liver injury. 4% increase in on-line gambling.

Alzheimer's & Dementia – 32% living with dementia report increased symptoms, apathy, resignation or "giving up"; ~60% show increase in behavioral & psychological symptoms; ~66% increase in stress-related symptoms in caregivers.

Eating Disorders – Overall increase in PTSDs, reduced access to support services.

Pregnancy & Parenthood – Reduction in personal human-contact support at all levels, leading to distress among mothers and infants. Reduction in confidence by expectant mothers and parents of newborns. Increased post-partum depression.

Sleep Disorders – 60% of people reporting worse sleep since lockdowns began, especially among young children.

Suicidal Behavior – Social isolation, anxiety, fear of contagion, uncertainty, chronic stress and economic difficulties are at work to increase depressive, anxious emotion, as well as substance abuse and psychiatric medications. Heightened suicidal risk among those with pre-existing conditions. Increased self-abuse and suicidal/self-harm thoughts, notably among women, low-income people, the unemployed and those with physical illness, mental disorders or Covid-19 diagnosis.

Mental Health Trends – Lockdown misery is similar to what is experienced by prisoners, no less than those sentenced by judges. Mental health care has largely deteriorated across the board. Nearly 20% of adults experience depression, double the pre-Covid-19 situation.

Domestic Violence/Child Abuse – 60% increase in battered women (Global). Schools and social services basically shut down along with primary & secondary health care, closures of daycare. Calls to UK hotlines reporting physical child abuse up by 32%. Increases in child sexual exploitation.

Table E: Physical Health[49]
Diseases and Conditions Made Worse by Covid-19
Hysteria, Lockdowns and Forced Masking: Reports are from peer-reviewed research in the UK unless otherwise noted

Cancers – Diagnostic declines from 19% to 72% in UK, 18,500 added deaths estimated within the 68 million UK population. [Author's NOTE: Extrapolated to USA population of 330 million (4.85 times more people), USA cancer deaths may have increased by ~90,000 additional over 2020.]

Cardiovascular disease (inclusive of heart disease and stroke) – UK: Excess deaths at home (+35%) and nursing homes/hospices (+32%) unrelated to Covid-19 infection. Increase in Out-of-Hospital Cardiac Arrest (56%). [Author's NOTE: The three average UK percentages is 41%. USA had 787,000 cardio-stroke deaths in 2011. Assuming half of those death numbers occurred out of hospital under Lockdown conditions (393,500), and using that 41% figure for a 2020 increase in figures, the USA may have experienced an additional 161,335 additional USA cardiovascular disease deaths for 2020. (USA data: *Heart Disease and Stroke Statistics*, American Heart/Stroke Association.)]

Children's health – Isolation misery, despair, malnutrition all on the rise. Globally ~30% reduction of essential nutrition in poverty nations. Closures of schools, loss of school sports exercise, lack of contact with peer-group friends, loss of romantic contacts, emotional trauma, increases in obesity, sleep, eating disorders.

Infectious diseases (other than Covid-19) – Globally: up to 400,000 extra TB deaths. Singapore: 37% increase is dengue fever cases.

Stroke – delays in treatment have exacerbated all aspects of recovery.

Surgery – delays have exacerbated all aspects of the original problems as well as the prospects of recovery.

To the above Tables we may add problems associated with increased poverty and homelessness due to lockdown economic disruptions. For example, a 1981 study "*Corporate Flight: The Causes and Consequences of Economic Dislocation*" by Bluestone et al.[50] indicated that "...a 1 percent increase in the unemployment rate will be associated with 37,000 deaths." Today, by that death toll per 1%, with a 40% increase in USA population from 1982 (232 mil.) to 2020 (330 mil.), and with a 6.7% unemployment rate, increased by 3.2% in 2020 from the pre-Covid era of 3.5%, that would compute to an estimated 165,760 additional *deaths by despair* in the USA for 2020, working its damage through all the paths and avenues mentioned above and below.[50] And *that is a minimal estimate*, given how lockdowns and economic ruin over 2020 was far worse than what was imagined by Bluestone, et al. in 1981.

From the UK also comes the following report, which would most surely reflect conditions in the USA, Canada and other Western democracies:

> "...alcohol-related deaths climbed to the highest in recorded history in the UK, with 5,460 deaths being logged between January and September alone... ...a dramatic increase in calls to the London Ambulance Service for suicide-related or attempted suicide reasons. Between March and November of last year, some 15,541 suicidal calls were logged by the service, up from 11,703 during the same time period the previous year. Lockdowns have severely impacted the mental health of children as well, with increasing numbers of children arriving at A&E hospitals after self-harming or overdosing on drugs... 'Children are a lost tribe in the pandemic. While they remain (for the most part) perplexingly immune to the health consequences of Covid-19, their lives and daily routines have been turned upside down.' ...children are increasingly suffering from anxiety, isolation, and boredom. 'Children in mental health crisis used to be brought to A&E about twice a week. Since the summer it's been more like once or twice a day. Some as young as 10 have cut themselves, taken overdoses, or tried to asphyxiate themselves'..." [51]

Additional published studies in peer-reviewed journals and private analysis confirm this awful situation produced by forced lockdowns and all associated with them:

* A study by the CDC indicated a USA 20% increase in the number of deaths due to accidental or deliberate drug overdoses, attributed to social isolation and financial hardship. Mostly that appears due to opioid addictions, and loss of funding for treatment programs. British Columbia experienced a 74% increase in overdose deaths over 2019.[52]

* An associated "epidemic of loneliness" also is occurring, with nearly half of young people showing signs of clinical depression, and 25% having suicidal thoughts.[53]

* Self-harm and substance abuse has increased among teens.[54]

* Canadian study: lockdowns created excess deaths, not Covid-19.[55]

* A study by John Pospichal: "Questions for Lockdown Apologists", published in late May 2020. He reviewed mortality figures for different states and nations during the early period of the Covid-19 crisis, showing lockdowns did not help to reduce deaths, but generally increased them. "...why did the virus...wait until lockdowns were imposed to suddenly start killing at levels which exceeded normal deaths?"[56]

* A study by Joel Smalley: "Dems COVID19 Lockdown Measures Causing Most Deaths", published on 27 June 2020 in *Principia Scientific International.* States governed by Democrats had a higher number of excess deaths than those governed by Republicans, which he attributed to the Democrat's stronger push for draconian lockdowns than the Republican's. "... the results of analysis of empirical data on mortality and counter-measure severity of all 50 US states, actually shows a statistically significant INCREASE in mortality associated with HIGHER degrees of counter-measure severity."[57]

* A study by T. Engelbrecht & C. Kohnlein: "COVID-19 (excess) mortalities: viral cause impossible – drugs with key role in about 200,000 extra deaths in Europe and the US alone."[58]

* A study by D.G. Rancourt et al. "Evaluation of the virulence of SARS-CoV-2 in France, from all-cause mortality 1946-2020". Conclusions:

"We are certain that this 'COVID-peak' is artificial... We suggest that: the unprecedented strict mass quarantine and isolation of both sick and healthy elderly people, together and separately, killed many of them, that this quarantine and isolation is the cause of the "COVID-peak" event that we have quantified, and that the medical mechanism is mainly via psychological stress and social isolation of individuals with health vulnerabilities. According to our calculations, this caused some 30.2K deaths in France in March and April 2020."[59]

It takes years for actual data to be recorded and reported on such factors, but the somewhat preliminary and anecdotal reports are indicative of *a gigantic unreported and conventionally ignored problem.*

Beyond all the above, there are the deleterious effects of forced masking upon respiration, and how they reduce oxygenation of the blood, and force one to constantly breathe in one's own oxygen-depleted exhalations. Masks not only contaminate the lungs with inhaled industrial micro-fibers and chemical vapors shed by various synthetic plastic materials, they also become a moist culture-dish for all kinds of bacterial and fungal growth that are also re-inhaled. They pose no obstacle for dry viral penetration, and allow infusion of absorbed droplets from talking, heavy breathing or sneezing, which are then also inhaled. Such masking also makes one more susceptible to accidents.

Here are the links to a four-part series from the *Primary Doctor Medical Journal,* on the health dangers and absence of protection from "masks".[60] A new malady called Mask-Induced Exhaustion Syndrome (MIES) has also been identified, from a meta-analysis of 65 different studies on short- and long-term mask wearing.[61]

Also important for a mention is the phenomenon of "long term Covid", where people get treated by conventional medicine but nevertheless persist with their symptoms, in spite of a subsequent negative PCR or antigen test. This may be due to the continued use of masks by that group of patients. "Long term Covid" may be no more complicated than the toxic effects of continued long-term mask-wearing and lockdowns. The above and similar articles on the *deadly pathological reactions* to the lockdowns are listed in a Supplementary Document.[14]

The effects of forced lockdowns, masking and inhuman anti-social distancing act like a wrecking ball upon the physical and emotional health and well-being of society, with a real and serious death count that is even greater than the 300,000+ deaths in 2020, and the 200,000+ deaths so far over 2021, all claimed to be due to Covid-19 alone. These increases due to lockdowns appear to be, in the final analysis, exactly what is being recorded and inaccurately blamed on "Covid-19".

In sum, we may estimate in Table F, as a by-product of all the forced lockdowns, masking, inhuman distancing and economic disruption related to Covid-19, the following incomplete and generalized death-counts:

Table F: *Rough Estimated* USA 2020 Deaths Created by Covid-19 Lockdowns, Masking and Destroyed Economy

Additional Cancer Deaths	89,725
Additional Heart/Pulmonary Disease Deaths	161,335
Additional Unemployment Deaths by Despair	165,760
Totals:	**416,820**

Table F only references those factors where a firm figure and percentage increase was available to make a calculation. As such they are probably *significantly low estimates.*

To Repeat: *A Possible Approximate 416,820 extra USA deaths due only to lockdowns, forced masking, inhuman distancing, economic ruin and related deaths by despair, may have occurred over 2020.*

Of course, each of the three Table F categories overlaps the others to some unknown degree, and many death-factors listed above in Tables D and E are not even included in the Table F limited analysis. So the actual net number of excess deaths due to forced lockdowns is presently unknown, being evaluated above *only* by reference to the small number of studies which actually came to my attention. It must be emphasized, this and the prior Table C figure of 250,000 excess deaths are *roughly estimated* short-lists of available data. The actual numbers *could be double that number.* For example, I have not been able to find actual data about increased suicides and drug overdoses, and many other factors, but assume those would fall into the "added unemployment" category. Are such assumptions valid? Whatever these preliminary figures indicate, several very great crimes can be identified in the analysis. These are presented in the Conclusions section of this book.

Basic Data on USA Annual Human Mortality

Assuming a deadly virus SARS-CoV-2 causing Covid-19 disease, and arguing from within that "official" paradigm, we should expect a pandemic to drive up the annual increase in all-cause deaths far more than the average annual increase in lives lost each year as from other causes, and thereby reduce overall life-expectancy for 2020. Using my own estimate of the 2020 year-end death tolls from all causes and extrapolating from provisional CDC data released on 26 December 2020, I could not believe the numbers made public by the CDC in early January 2021. There were two major "data dumps" contained within them, both of which appeared quite suspicious.

In addition to updating its Covid-19 death totals, the CDC and its subsidiary National Center for Health Statistics (NCHS) added several hundred thousand all-cause deaths into their 2020 year-end calculations. Here in Figure 13 are three screen shots from the CDC websites, for their Dec. 19, Dec. 26, 2020, and Jan. 2, 2021 calculations. A summary of the numbers is given in Table G.

The rise in all-cause deaths in the last week of 2020 was a giant number – 269,249 – five times what might be expected by the usual prior weeks of more gradual increases. Another factor is how in early January

2021, the Covid-19 death numbers rose by an additional ~87,000 – from the reported 313,171 to a nice round media-announced 400,000 – two astonishing data-dumps within a few days.

This becomes all the more acute when reviewed over the prior decade. Table H below provides the all-cause death and annual increase death numbers going back to 2010. There is a trend of rising annual all-cause death numbers with an annual increase in each subsequent year reflecting steadily expanding population growth. Life Expectancy remains about the same for the decade, at around 78.5 to 78.9 years, the number for 2020 being estimated without Covid-19. The *annual increases* in all-cause deaths are also variable over the decade with an unexpected minima of 15,633 in 2019, a maxima of 86,212 in 2015, and of course 317,075 in 2020 – with an overall average annual rise from 2010 to 2019 of 44,806. The numbers presented here for 2020 are provisional through the end of the year, using CDC and other data sources as referenced.

At first, I could not accept the CDC's two year end "data dump" numbers, of either the 317,075 annual increase in all-cause deaths, or the quick early January 2021 increase of 87,000 Covid-19 deaths, nearly overnight. Today, I accept the actual year-end death totals. However, two separate major errors are revealed:

Figure 13: Year-End Changes in CDC All-Cause and Covid-19 Data[62]

19 Dec. 2020	26 Dec. 2020	2 Jan. 2021
All Deaths involving COVID-19 (U07.1)[1] — Deaths from All Causes	All Deaths involving COVID-19 (U07.1)[1] — Deaths from All Causes	All Deaths involving COVID-19 (U07.1)[1] — Deaths from All Causes
291,757 2,851,438	301,679 2,902,664	313,171 3.171,913

Notice the increase in Covid-19 and all-cause deaths over this two week period:

Table G: Week of	Rise in Covid-19 Deaths	Rise in All-Cause Deaths
19 to 26 Dec.	9,922	51,226
26 Dec.20 to 2 Jan.21	11,492	**269,249**

Error 1: The Covid-19 death numbers are a misinterpretation (or misrepresentation) of deaths by multiple comorbidities, for the simple reason of their showing up as "positive results" on highly inaccurate PCR and Antigen tests, or by equally inaccurate clinical diagnoses in hospitals. Financial motivations as discussed on page 39 also exist.

Error 2: The elevated death figures for 2020 in the "Covid-19" category, inclusive within the "All Causes" category, are the consequences of lockdowns, forced masking, inhuman distancing, economic ruin and *deaths by despair.* These were deliberately imposed upon a panicked and frightened population, at the point of a policeman's gun.

Covid-19 death counts appear in reality to be an *artificial diagnostic category* for those who actually died of the other-cause comorbidities, diseases and disorders which have been significantly intensified over 2020 due to the lockdown hysteria. There also are cases where a person died in a traffic accident, or was shot in a robbery, with the death certificate reading "Covid-19". Less frequently do we hear about the massive inaccuracies of the "laboratory testing" methods, or the significantly large number of deaths due solely to economic ruin and isolation despair, where lockdowns, masking and economic disintegration have their own "comorbidities", driving people into an early grave.

Table H: Number of People Dying Each Year in the USA, All Causes, with Annual Increases From the Prior Year

Year	All-Cause Deaths[1]	Annual Increase	"Covid-19" Deaths	Life Expect.[2]
2010:	2,468,435			78.49y
2011:	2,515,458	47,023		78.64y
2012:	2,543,279	27,821		78.79y
2013:	2,596,993	53,714		78.94y
2014:	2,626,418	29,425		78.91y
2015:	2,712,630	86,212		78.89y
2016:	2,774,248	61,618		78.86y
2017:	2,813,503	39,255		78.84y
2018:	2,839,205	25,702		78.81y
2019:	2,854,838	15,633		78.87y
2020:[3]	**3,171,913[3]**	**317,075[3]**	**313,171[4]**	**78.93y[2]**

1. https://www.cdc.gov/nchs/products/nvsr.htm "Deaths: Leading Causes for (year)" 2. Life Expectancy & Other Data. *For 2020,* estimated without Covid-19: https://www.macrotrends.net/countries/USA/united-states/life-expectancy 3. Provisional 2020 data from 1 Jan 2020 to 2 Jan.2021.   4. or 400,000 ?? https://www.cdc.gov/nchs/nvss/vsrr/covid_weekly/index.htm

These last minute data dumps amplified my own alarm after nearly a year of growing suspicion, given how nearly every source from government and mass media had been steadily blaring horns and beating loud drums, as if to deliberately drive a herd of elk over a cliff – to push people into even more panic and hysteria, so that the public would meekly accept the lockdowns and forced masking as some kind of "scientific-medical" necessity. To "save lives"! Or "for the children"! Our "top leaders" in government, media and medicine demanded such harsh measures without any mention of, or concern for the consequences of their actions!

Also suspicious is how graphics on the CDC's "Covid Weekly" websites confined their weekly data analyses to the years 2017 through 2020, thereby avoiding comparisons to the high mortality years of 2015 to 2016 as shown in Table H above. Is this because 2020 "P&I" and/or "PIC" comorbidities as redefined into the Covid-19 category, are not so different from the high death numbers of 2015-2016? Too many in the medical profession, and in government and media, apparently do not know about, or choose to believe that economic ruin, prisoner-types of lockdowns, or death by despair are a fantasy, are not solid and real traumas that kill people. And so they simply never mention them.

A graphic seen in Figure 14 is a case in point, presenting the all-cause deaths from early 2017 to early 2021. It is taken from the Euromomo website,[63] exposing additional suspicious factors. *Firstly*, the graphic correctly shows relatively accurately the seasonal December-January Northern Hemisphere wintertime aspect, with the major increases in deaths for all years shown as marked with a "W". Euromomo did not mention this obvious fact which drives death rates higher, all by itself.

Secondly, the Figure 14 baseline does not accurately reflect the annual increases, from one year to the next. The area under the peaks, above the baseline for 2020 appears as only 10 times that of 2019, and 5 times that of 2018. The peaks for 2020 should in fact be far greater in size, around double of what is shown.

Third, the years going back to 2015 had incrementally higher all-cause and annual increase deaths as shown in the numerical insert for Figure 14, but the graph only starts sometime in the 12th week of 2017, not showing the early winter months of 2017. Had the graph been extended back to 2014, it would have revealed that the peaks of 2020 were not so unusual. To therefore attribute the 2020 peaks as "excess deaths due to Covid-19" which include the giant numbers as previously given, cannot be true. Or if so, in this graphic, Covid19 would be no worse than an ordinary year with a lot of influenza and pneumonia.

Fourth, this graphic is supposed to inform the viewer how 2020 death numbers were so much higher than prior years, to validate the Covid-19 pandemic theory. Showing only three years of prior data is insufficient.

And *Fifth*, note how the ordinate vertical scale of the graph does not start at zero, but rather around 40,000. If it had started at zero, the graph would either have been twice as tall, or compressed down wherein the peaks for all years would be greatly diminished and not look so "scary".

There is a wonderful small book titled *How to Lie With Statistics* by Darrel Huff.[64] It was required reading in the university when I was younger. Nevertheless, it should be apparent to everyone how the truncated data selection and exaggeration of the data curves are primary methods of deceiving people, without "outright lying". Perhaps this is all simple coincidence and not planned deception, but who knows?

Figure 14: Euromomo Graphic[63]

Total Deaths		Annual Increase
Year	All Causes	from Prior Year
2015:	2,712,630	86,212
2016:	2,774,248	61,618
2017:	2,813,503	39,255
2018:	2,839,205	25,702
2019:	2,854,838	15,633
2020:	3,171,913	317,075 or 400,000 ??

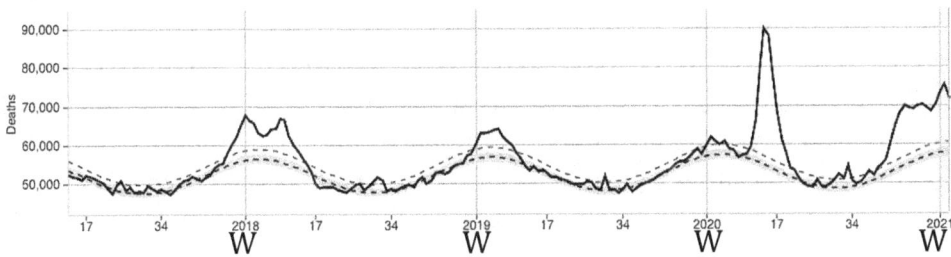

— Pooled deaths   Normal range ···· Baseline ···· Substantial increase   Corrected for delay in registration

All ages

USA Covid-19 and All-Cause Death Counts by Age Group

Tables I and J below add to our concerns about the CDC data and Covid-19 pandemic in a more quantitative manner, revealing how the *Covid-19* and *all-cause* death numbers by age group, transformed into percentages of the totals of those two categories, show *nearly identical distributions of deaths among the elderly*, 65 years and older. This makes no sense if there is truly a serious pandemic of a new infectious virus that preferentially attacks the respiratory systems of the elderly, thereby killing them.

For example, Covid-19 disease does not affect young children to any extent, given their natural immunity. That curious aspect is affirmed in the Table I data, presented below with a full year of 2020 data (1 Jan 2020 to 2 Jan 2021) directly from a CDC/NCHS website. Covid-19 is also supposed to be killing significantly higher percentages of the elderly than other causes. However the Table I data does not affirm that to any significance. While the 313,171 Covid-19 deaths constitute 9.87% of the 3,171,913 all-cause deaths for 2020, this increase is overwhelmingly confined to the four oldest Covid-19 death categories, of 55-64 years, 65-74 years, 75-84 years and 85+ years, where pre-existing comorbidities are highest and PCR misidentifications are most abundant. In the groups from birth up to 54 years of age, fewer deaths are attributed to Covid-19 relative to all-causes, a factor I have never seen emphasized elsewhere. When taking those deaths, or lack of deaths, in the younger age groups into consideration, the overall total USA 2020 "Covid-19 excess deaths" drops dramatically, to 4,866 persons.

After reducing each age-group death number into a percentage of its column total, then extracting the difference in those percentages (%Cov minus %All = %Diff) across each age group, and then converting the differences in those percentages into a proportion of the age-group Covid death numbers (Covid-19 Number times %Diff), the numbers of excess deaths for each category were extracted. *Given how the Covid-19 and all-cause deaths in the vulnerable elderly groups are nearly identical, it fully undermines the claim of a new and deadly Covid-19 viral pandemic.*

In some cases, fewer people died in a given age-specific Covid-19 category than would be expected by comparison to the all-cause death numbers. In other cases, notably the elderly groups, a slightly higher number of death numbers occurred – but not by much. The total number of excess deaths in the Covid-19 category, above the baseline percentages created by all other causes, was calculated to be 4,866 – an astonishing low number given all the panic, hysteria, lockdowns, economic destruction, etc. that government, medicine and media claim are "necessary".

That number of 4,866 excess deaths in Table I works out to be around 13 extra deaths per day, for the entire USA. *Thirteen.* I also ran those numbers through an Excel program, and a second time as seen in Table J, using slightly different assumptions, just to be certain of my methodology and numbers.

For Table I, the figure of 3.17 million all-cause deaths includes the total Covid-19 death counts. That being the case, fully accurate proportional calculations must remove the Covid-19 counts from the all-cause counts. I therefore made a new calculation in Table J, where the Covid-19 death numbers for each age group were subtracted from the same age categories of all-causes deaths. That revised Table J provides a more robust calculation, *assuming the original CDC data is itself robust, which is an open question.* Table J indicates 5,399 total 2020 US excess deaths, a bit higher than as seen in Table I, but hardly significant in terms of overall determinations. *The 5,399 deaths are equal to about 15 deaths per day, for the entire USA.*

Two different calculations have been provided, using different iterations of the publicly-announced CDC Covid-19 and all-cause death numbers for the whole of 2020. No matter how these numbers are reviewed or calculated, in either Table I or J, the final annual excess USA deaths are extremely low by the standard expectations of a raging pandemic requiring massive lockdowns, and justifying state-enforced totalitarian measures. *No amount of nit-picking, to change the numbers by even hundreds or thousands of quanta, alters that outcome.*

Below is a final Table K, which summarizes the conclusions from the Tables I and J (on the following two pages).

Table K: Excess Deaths for 2020:

Total Deaths:	All Causes	Covid-19 Deaths (?)		
		Num	%	Excess Deaths
Table I	3,171,913	313,171	9.87%	4,866
Table J	2,858,742	313,171	10.9%	5,399
		Average:	**10.4%**	**5,132**

Tables I and J included the CDC's Annual Increase of 317,075 all-cause deaths (from Table H), but not the additional early January 2021 data increase of approximately 87,000 deaths, to justify the media-reported 400,000 number for Covid-19 deaths. However, neither of those data-

Table I: USA 2020 Deaths by Covid-19 & All Causes, by Age Group, with Covid-19 deaths included in the All Cause death number[65]

1 Jan.20 to 2 Jan.21	Covid-19 Number	%Cov[1]	All Causes	US Deaths %All[2]	%Diff.[3]	US Excess Deaths[4]
All Ages =>	313,171	9.87%	3,171,913			
Under 1 year	32	0.01%	17,750	0.56%	-0.55%	0
1–4 years	19	0.006%	3,276	0.10%	-0.097%	0
5–14 years	54	0.017%	5,247	0.17%	-0.148%	0
15–24 years	494	0.16%	33,598	1.06%	-0.9%	-4
25–34 years	2,129	0.68%	68,807	2.17%	-1.49%	-32
35–44 years	5,559	1.78%	97,549	3.1%	-1.3%	-72
45–54 years	14,963	4.8%	178,444	5.63%	-0.85%	-127
55–64 years	37,235	11.9%	412,045	13%	-1.1%	-410
65–74 years	66,745	21.3%	630,360	19.9%	+1.44%	+961
75–84 years	85,925	27.4%	770,041	24.3%	+3.16%	+2,715
85 years +	100,016	31.9%	954,796	30.1%	+1.83%	+1,835

Total Covid-19 Excess Deaths Above All Causes: 4,866

https://www.cdc.gov/nchs/nvss/vsrr/covid_weekly/index.htm
Jan.2, 2021 update, remained posted on CDC webpage through 7 Jan.
  1. Percent of deaths in each Covid-19 age group relative to Covid-19 "All Ages" total deaths; numerical age and all-age total data copied directly from 26 Dec. CDC update.
  2. Percent of deaths in each All Causes age group relative to All Causes "All Ages" total deaths.
  3. Percent difference, %Cov minus %All.
  4. Excess Death Number Extrapolation from %Diff by age group, of claimed Covid-19 deaths.

Table J: USA 2020 Deaths by Covid-19 & All Causes, by Age Group, with Covid-19 deaths subtracted from the All Cause death number[65]

1 Jan.20 to 2 Jan.21	Covid-19 Number	%Cov[1]	US All Causes Minus Cov	%All[2]	%Diff.[3]	US Excess Deaths[4]
All Ages =>	313,171	10.9%	2,858,742			
Under 1 year	32	0.01%	17,718	0.62%	-0.61%	0
1–4 years	19	0.006%	3,257	0.11%	-0.1%	0
5–14 years	54	0.017%	5,193	0.18%	-0.16%	0
15–24 years	494	0.16%	33,104	1.16%	-1%	-5
25–34 years	2,129	0.7%	66,678	2.3%	-1.6%	-35
35–44 years	5,559	1.8%	91,990	3.2%	-1.4%	-80
45–54 years	14,963	4.8%	163,481	5.7%	-0.94%	-141
55–64 years	37,235	12%	374,810	13%	-1.2%	-455
65–74 years	66,745	21.3%	563,615	19.7%	+1.6%	+1,066
75–84 years	85,925	27.4%	684,116	23.9%	+3.5%	+3,013
85 years +	100,016	31.9%	854,780	29.9%	+2%	+2,036

Total Covid-19 Excess Deaths Above All Causes: 5,399

https://www.cdc.gov/nchs/nvss/vsrr/covid_weekly/index.htm
All Causes deaths are minus the Covid-19 number for each age group.
Same reference notes as for the adjacent Table I.

dumps, nor other variations in data or calculations mattered at all, in terms of providing a significantly different outcome in computed excess deaths due to Covid-19. The numbers do not lie.

The official CDC data on total Covid-19 and all-cause deaths, segregated into different age groups, shows approximately the same percentage of deaths, with total claimed Covid-19 excess deaths averaging 5,132 for 2020. Or one can choose to use the higher number from Table J, of 5,399 excess deaths. It does not matter. That higher number works out to be around 15 deaths per day, for the whole USA, for all of 2020. These figures for the excess deaths due to Covid-19 are extremely low, from 13 to 15 daily US deaths, even lower than the CDC's own post-February figure of "over 5%" without comorbidities,[30] which computes to around 15,658 deaths over 2020. Or Ealy, et al's above-mentioned 6% of Covid-19 deaths without comorbidities,[8] which computed to 18,790 deaths for the year, or 52 deaths per day, over all 50 states. *Again, that is about 1 death per state per day.*

None of these computations provide justifications for such massive governmental and medical-media panic-peddling, with lockdowns and other very deadly totalitarian interferences in the health, income and lives of ordinary people.

One must keep in mind how respiratory illness has always been a major factor in the deaths of elderly people. Those over 65 years of age constitute about 88% of all cases of pneumonia and influenza. They are also a vulnerable group heavily hit with *death by despair*, and who succumb to whatever comorbidity factors they are afflicted with. *Emotional anxiety, despair* and comorbidity factors overshadow everything that is claimed for the SARS-CoV-2 killer super-virus.

Given the serious inaccuracy of Covid-19 PCR/Antigen test kits, the re-definitions of pneumonia, influenza and other comorbidities as "Covid-19" (eg, "P&I" and "PIC" confusions, discussed above), and the fact that the majority of claimed Covid-19 cases and deaths occur during wintertime cold-damp conditions, we can expect the misdiagnosed and inflated Covid-19 category to be biased towards inclusion of more people in the older age groups, whether or not they were truly infected with a new and deadly virus. This is aside from the financial or virus-ideology motivations for hospital administrators to favorably place Covid-19 on death certificates rather than the comorbidities which actually killed their patients. Such factors all trend for *a biased and unscientific selection of deceased elderly patients into the Covid-19 category.*

These data, as used in my Tables I and J, obtained from official CDC sources but reviewed in a different manner than usual, coupled with evidence of Covid-19's non-exclusive symptomology overlapping with many other diseases and disorders, demolish the claims of a severe Covid-19 pandemic demanding "emergency-panic-lockdown" reactions.

Covid-19 Death Data Inconsistencies Identified by Genevieve Briand... *Censored by Johns Hopkins*

In mid-November 2020, the study "Covid-19 Deaths: A Look at U.S. Data" was presented at a webinar[66] by Dr. Genevieve Briand, Assistant Director of the Applied Economics Program at Johns Hopkins University. Briand reviewed all-cause and Covid-19 US deaths up to that November date. Her webinar was then summarized in an article by Yanni Gu, posted on Nov. 22 to *The Johns Hopkins News-Letter* (JHNL)[67] as "Published by the Students of Johns Hopkins since 1896". The *News-Letter* article reviewed Briand's findings which revealed an over-counting of 2020 Covid-19 deaths that could not be reconciled with the available all-cause deaths, probably due to confusions of Covid-19 with other diseases, as I also concluded independently. The Briand/Gu article stimulated a controversy and was then "retracted" (censored) from the JHNL four days later by its editors, for the reason it "has been used to support dangerous inaccuracies that minimize the impact of the pandemic."

The reactions of the editors at JHNL was a clear case of "Don't confuse us with the facts, our minds are already made up!" After reviewing the CDC data, Briand's analysis and conclusions were anything but inaccurate: As CDC-confirmed Covid-19 deaths increased during the April 2020 peak, most all other causes of death declined, indicating a shifting of other diseases into the Covid-19 category, as I concluded above. Her closing webinar statement was apropos:

"We don't know if a death is from Covid first, or a [different] condition. How are we to best address it? If someone has a heart condition and is over 50, what is the best way to prevent death by Covid-19 or heart attack? Is it to isolate myself, or to exercise? When I see the poster of the CDC of physically inactive people sitting on a bench, with the self-distancing... should you exercise, is that going to be a better way to engage and interact? If you are depressed your immune system goes down... the question is, what is the best way to fight [disease]? To isolate yourself? Or to be happy and meet people, and get out and exercise. And live." (G. Briand, starting around 1:04:45)[66]

The original webpage for the Briand/Gu article was quickly replaced by a statement by the JHNL editors, rationalizing their censorship.[67] A PDF of the original article was provided, but with the obscuring banner, "Retracted by The News-Letter" contemptuously plastered across every page.[68]

My Tables I and J above provided a similar form of analysis, extended to the end of 2020, wherein I independently observed the same data inconsistencies, and came to similar conclusions.

Alarmist Reporting on Death Counts

On December 22, just before Christmas 2020, the Associated Press (AP) released an alarmist report that the year would end with from 3 to 3.2 million all-cause deaths, *a figure suggestively blamed on Covid-19, complete with a photograph from the 1918 influenza epidemic.* This hysterical report, attributed to the CDC but without any confirming reference, was quickly picked up by nearly every major newspaper and media outlet in the USA, and some overseas. Those alarming numbers were blasted out as top headlines, as if they were all Covid-19 *deaths*, but with little clarification. Grim-faced broadcast media stars seized the opportunity to further drive up the panic and hysteria.[69]

Within a few days, around the end of 2020, the sum of 400,000 USA Covid-19 deaths was also being circulated in the national and international media. This merely added to the fear and panic that was already being promoted by medical and government health bureaucrats. Power-drunk politicians also weighed in. For example, the CDC Covid Tracker website screamed out misleading full-year *cumulative numbers* for the USA in a manner conflating "cases" with deaths. They posted in large text "OVER 17 MILLION TOTAL CASES", "1.6 MILLION CASES IN LAST 7 DAYS" followed by "312,636 TOTAL DEATHS". By early January 2021, it was "20.5 MILLION CASES" and "350,644 DEATHS".[70] A NY Times website, mentioned above in my Table C regarding death/case ratios in the different states, continued promoting hysteria, with numerous state "cases" data graphs that were 7-10 times higher than the actual deaths, the latter of which were not shown on their graphics. Such alarmist reporting was to deliberately scare and mislead people to conclude that the "cases" were the primary important factor, as they pondered just what the risk of death might be for themselves and family.

Even if those media numbers were accurate, the way they were reported in a *cumulative total manner*, created the false impression among ordinary people that 17 or 20 million Americans were dying or would soon be dead from claimed Covid-19. The Johns Hopkins University Covid-19 tracker webpage was similar, with big fonts... 85+ million... 20 million... all that was missing were multiple exclamation points. ("Horreurs!!!!")[71]

The WHO Covid-19 website did the same with global numbers: "85 Million Confirmed Cases of Covid-19, Including 1.8 million deaths."[72]

The above statements were announced as the top item on their websites, without clarification that the overwhelming number of "cases" were asymptomatic people who were not sick or infectious. Or that the dying and dead were very old and fragile, suffering over years from multiple other diseases and conditions, and were already approaching the end of their lives. Or that many died at home or in the emergency room, and were hence PCR tested *post-mortem*, where the real causes of deaths were ignored in favor of claimed "Covid-19", to drive up the numbers. They also did not clarify that the "millions" figures did NOT represent the number of people actually dying in their local towns, counties or states. By such methods they deliberately fanned the flames of public panic and hysteria. Similarly, when searching on Google for "Corona viruses", you are automatically directed to page after page of hysterical Covid fear-porn. Everything was, and still is organized to increase panic and anxiety, not to calm people down.

As I stated above: *The USA never experienced such crowded hospitals as seen in the Chinese videos, with people dropping dead in the street. Nobody was burying their neighbors either, no trucks slowly moving through the streets calling to "bring out your dead", even as major media and government "experts" fanned the flames of hysteria as if this was such a situation.*

How could the average person *not* be deeply frightened by such irrational and unnecessary displays, to include *cumulative total numbers since January 2020, going up, Up and UP,* rather than the actual lowering trends, as I've demonstrated. In 2021, as I write this, new Covid-19 numbers are being added into those of 2020, with claims of "new strains" or variants of Covid-19. More contrived panic. How can ordinary people not believe that their very lives and those of their children are in severe danger unless they lock down and shelter at home, with forced masking, etc., especially if that's all they hear or see?

And that brings us to the alarming phenomenon of *how mainstream news media and internet have conspired to censor and personally destroy by slander, the voices of independent scientists and doctors who oppose the lockdowns and forced masking (and in 2021, the vaccine hysteria).* The massive censorship exerted today by mainstream media, and by the internet billionaires running Google, Facebook, Twitter, YouTube and the like, suggests a deliberate cover-up of all the facts that run counter to such panic-inducing official pronouncements. The true goal appears to be, *to erase any publicly-uttered opinion contrary to the WHO or CDC, so that ordinary people won't hear much of anything beyond what the new Medical Police State, or Pharmaceutical Big Brother, is telling them.*

As previously noted, such scare-talk causes additional deaths due to fear, anxiety, panic, lockdowns and economic devastation, being the probable real cause of the high 2020/2021 death numbers, as previously stated. And how many of those deaths are misidentified as "deaths due to Covid-19"? *Covid hysteria* indirectly contributed to all of them.

Many professionals have stepped forward to challenge the claims of the Covid-19 "pandemic" – as in the thousands of brave physicians and other public health scientists who signed the *Great Barrington Declaration*, or the members of the *America's Front-Line Doctors, and Association of American Physicians and Surgeons.* Another group challenging the massive lockdown terrorism, and the bogus claim that "only a vaccine will save us" is led by Robert F. Kennedy Jr., the *Children's Health Defense.* A more comprehensive list of these and similar organizations, with weblinks to their websites, is given at the end of this book.

ALL of these groups, and many others, are restricted or erased from Facebook, Twitter, YouTube, etc., their voices muzzled as in a totalitarian state. These dissenting physicians, scientists and others take a great risk of being publicly slandered, or to lose their medical licenses, university posts, research funding, etc., with their websites censored and sometimes suffering criminal prosecutions thereafter. This is so, even as the majority of professionals have willingly, or due to threats and fear, accepted the deadly status quo over the health and well-being of the public. While many are innocents in this deadly affair, most of the health professionals and scientists at the top levels of universities, institutionalized medicine and government are doubly complicit. They have remained tone-deaf or silent, even while other's wrong-headed conclusions gave license and ammunition to socially destructive politicians. Those politicians then bark out anti-constitutional "dictates" for never-ending lockdowns, towards formation of a literal Medical Police State. ***Where does it end?***

Problems in Medical Diagnosis, Ethics, and the Suppression of Scientific-Medical Dissent

The medical profession has a long history of suppressing its own members when they stray from consensus ideas. This becomes deadly when concealment of medical blunders has taken place. In the mid 1800s, Ignatz Semmelweis discovered the cause of childbed fever in the doctor's own unwashed hands, as they went from disease-ridden wards or the autopsy room, directly to giving pelvic exams to pregnant and laboring women. Thousands of women and infants perished. Semmelweis observed this happening, and demanded the physicians under his direction wash their hands with chloride of lime, to prevent infectious germs from being carried into the pregnant women's wards. By this simple step, childbed fever, or puerperal fever, was eventually ended. For his discovery, Semmelweis was viciously attacked and slandered, fired from one hospital post to another, and eventually locked up in a mental asylum by a conspiracy of his peers. In that case, it was the medical profession's denial of the germ theory of disease, and of their own dirty, contaminated hands, which led to massive deaths of women and their babies.

Another official medical horror show occurred during the 20th Century in Nazi Germany. It was medical doctors who organized to set up the first euthanasia "hospitals" of the Nazi Third Reich, where deformed and retarded children were among the first to be exterminated, thereafter followed by the disabled elderly and criminals in prison camps – the "useless eaters". Soon enough, political prisoners and "unclean, disease-infested and genetically unfit undesirables" were killed, a curse hurled upon Jews, Gypsies, Slavs, Serbs and others. They were rounded up by SS troops, but examined and segregated as to who would live, and who would die, by white-coated medical doctors. The medical doctors also performed horrible experiments on prisoners, including children. They perfected the use of Zyklon-B poison gas for exterminations, and monitored death-camp guards to weed out those "too soft" to undertake the murderous tasks demanded of them. Medical students were sent to the death camps also, to "observe and learn". But most of that ugly genocidal history of relatively recent modern medicine isn't taught anymore, isn't spoken about in polite company, isn't in the textbooks. Like the contrary evidence undermining Covid-19 theory, it is all censored out. (See Henry Friedlander's well-referenced and shocking book "The Origins of Nazi Genocide: From Euthanasia to the Final Solution."[73])

Similar barbarisms were also undertaken in WW2 by Imperial Japanese medical experts, using civilians and war prisoners for horrible medical experiments, testing black plague germs and other biological weapons on them. The same biological warfare agents were then unleashed upon Chinese civilians, killing hundreds of thousands, all with the imprimatur of "medical expertise".

While comparisons of modern medicine to war criminals may seem unfair, medicine has always partnered with those in power, in both free or slave nations. Genetic theory was historically abused to label some people as disposably "inferior". Today in the USA, it is abused to seriously mutilate perfectly healthy women by "preventive mastectomy", or merged with superstitions to justify full castration of the sexual organs of young people suffering from socially-induced gender dysphoria. In these cases, there is no scientifically defendable evidence or proofs to substantiate the mutilations. Sexual misery, depression, drug addictions and suicides are known consequences. Psychiatry has also been politicized.

After firstly rejecting the idea, modern medicine accepts the existence of infectious microbes, but additional medical disasters have subsequently taken root by stretching the germ theory beyond all rational limits. So-called "hiding" or "slow viruses" are a case in point. These were proposed as disease mechanisms starting in the 1980s, with the *Acquired* Immune Deficiency Syndrome (AIDS), when physicians ignored the original "acquired" environmental-behavioral component and embraced a viral causation even when it could not be definitively isolated or proven. The "infectious HIV" theory spread panic, claiming that while you got infected today, symptoms for AIDS would not appear for 10 years or more. And when you did get sick, the symptoms imitated over 60 different "indicator diseases" – as with today's "viral comorbidities".

PCR tests were developed for HIV, which were no more accurate than the modern PCR tests are for Covid-19. Toxic pharmaceuticals such as azidothymidine (AZT) killed unknown thousands of people in the AIDS years, leaving many major open questions about the legitimacy of the infectious HIV theory. Critics of the slow-hiding virus theory, such as top virologist Peter Duesberg,[74] were attacked and isolated, subjected to censorship of their articles in scientific publications, and punished or "weeded-out" from the universities or medical institutions. Critics of "infectious HIV" theory were vilified in the mainstream media as "AIDS deniers", with open calls by HIV "experts" to have them imprisoned to shut them up. Few people today even know about the HIV controversies due to continuing censorship.

Today, with Covid-19, a similar censorship and vilification of dissenters and critics is occurring. Beyond the excessive cycling of PCR methods yielding many false positives, as discussed above, it appears certain that diagnoses of Covid-19 have the same problems of poor documentation and isolation proofs, and lack of clear causality as occurred previously with respect to AIDS and HIV.

Covid-19 cases and deaths, conventionally attributed to an infectious virus SARS-CoV-2, are more easily understood as true *influenza, pneumonia, congestive heart disease, and other maladies that are worsened during wintertime epochs of cold temperatures and moisture.* Beyond winter chills, other climate factors are at work driving up influenza and pneumonia, as in India or Brazil, hot-humid regions where incessant rain and flooding during summertime monsoons affects large tropical populations. Or elsewhere, dry dusty or pollen-rich atmospheres trigger additional respiratory distress. Under all those conditions, lung and heart functions of elderly people with other existing diseases and disorders, are exacerbated. *Such respiratory conditions were, prior to Covid-19, diagnosed according to presenting symptoms.* Today, however, biochemical PCR and antigen tests are generally the diagnostic procedure of choice. People get tested, and if positive, the physician may "treat the test", not the patient.

Even before PCR tests, medical errors developed when certain diseases were prematurely attributed to infectious microbes. One example was the pellagra epidemic in the USA, and another, the SMON epidemic primarily in Japan. Physicians assumed these were infectious disorders given how they occurred among groups of people in close proximity, as in families or other population groups, but without questioning the unproven, dogmatically-believed basic assumptions about those diseases.

Pellagra is characterized by fatigue, diarrhea, dermatitis, open sores and dementia, culminating in death. It afflicted families and populations in the rural US Southern states. Starting in the early 1900s and running into the 1940s, some 3 million people were affected, with over 100,000 deaths. For reasons of close proximity it was assumed to be an infectious disorder, caused by an as-yet undefined microbe. "Pellagrites" were frequently shunned, and due to dementia were placed in long-term mental hospitals. Pellagra was eventually found to be caused by poor diets lacking in Vitamin B3 (niacin) and tryptophan, as is typical of corn-based diets in poverty regions with low dietary milk, fresh fruits and vegetables. Physician Joseph Goldberger made that discovery in 1915, after bringing pellagra patients back to health by dietary changes and vitamin supplementation. He also proved pellagra could not be infectious by undertaking deliberate injection experiments. Many years passed, with additional deaths, before his findings were widely accepted.

SMON disease (Subacute Myelo-Optico-Neuropathy) had a similar but shorter epoch, appearing as a tourist disorder primarily in Japan from 1955 through 1970. It was characterized by increasing diarrhea, weight loss, disabling paralysis, blindness and death. Around 100,000 SMON deaths occurred in Japan, with more around the world, being attributed to an unknown infectious virus. SMON was later understood as the side-effect of the abundantly-prescribed anti-diarrhea medicine *clioquinol*. Once clioquinol was banned and its manufacturer Ciba-Geigy abandoned its production in 1985, SMON disease disappeared globally. SMON was first identified as an iatrogenic disorder by physician Olle Hansson of Norway, who campaigned against clioquinol, meeting stiff opposition from conventional medicine. The case of SMON not only duplicated the problem of a too-quick attribution of a deadly disease to a microbe, but also ignored more obvious signs of toxic reactions to favored "medicines".

The skepticism against Goldberger's and Hansson's findings, and the personal opposition they were greeted with, is repeated today in a far worse manner by highly organized and well-funded Big Medicine. Dissenting physicians and scientists may suffer vilification, censoring and silencing if they dare challenge the government-backed "official truth" about Covid-19. Some political totalitarians already advocate detention camps for Covid-19 dissenters, for those who refuse to be vaccinated, or who are "disobedient" to medical authority. Similar demands to lock up dissenters were heard during the AIDS years, to silence critics of the conventional "infectious HIV" theory of AIDS. They were called "AIDS Deniers", just as today the term "Covid Deniers" has become a popular curse, to demonize critics as if they were Nazi Holocaust deniers.

A very good accounting of the pharmaceutical industry's profiteering and deadly suppression of dissent by cooperative mainstream media and conventional medicine is found in the excellent book *Racketeering In Medicine*.[75] And while a bit out of date, my article on "Suppression of Dissent in Science and Medicine", gives numerous examples and further citations on that subject.[76] The historical examples recounted in those materials, for which justice was never found, laid the foundations for what we observe today with censorship of criticisms of Covid-19.

Today the virologists' errors are compounded by medicine, with often ineffective but toxic and expensive drugs against Covid-19, or the influenza and pneumonia which defines it, while at the same time working to deny and make illegal effective and inexpensive out-of-patent medicines.

Banned and Slandered, but Effective Remedies

Examples of the banned but effective and economical medicines include hydroxychloroquine, an anti-malaria and anti-lupus drug widely available in many parts of the world, notably in Africa, where it can be purchased over the counter. It is an effective remedy for Covid-19 symptoms as well, especially when combined with zinc supplements.[77] Another remedy is high-dose vitamin C therapy, firstly advocated by Nobel-Prize winner Linus Pauling in the 1980s, but severely attacked by American medicine given its efficacy against colds, influenza, and cancer. Many physicians use it today for lung-distressed patients, as an IV-drip of 20 to 40 grams per day. Usually only a few days of such therapy is necessary for significant recovery. One can also home-treat with high-dose vitamin C (powdered calcium ascorbate is best, dissolved in water).[78] Combined with high-dose vitamin D therapy it is very beneficial against lung-heart problems, something which modern medicine deprives people of by promoting lockdown madness that keeps people away from sunlight.[79] Ivermectin or azitheromycin are other out-of-patent economical medicines proving effective against breathing disorders, also showing benefits to those with a Covid-19 diagnosis who are truly ill, whether it is factually influenza, pneumonia or something else.[80] Furthermore, the use of zinc or silver-ion supplements or lozenges are helpful. Nebulized hydrogen peroxide can also be a natural remedy approach for home treatment, and an alternative to questionable hospitalization.

Mainstream media and medicine denies or avoids mention of these home-based treatments due to their ideological and financial alliances with Big Pharma and BioTech, who advertise heavily in science and medical journals, and on public media. The mainstream media then supports only the most orthodox and conventional of treatments, lying and misreporting on alternatives. One motivation behind the suppression of inexpensive and effective medicines or home-remedies is the big push for vaccines against Covid-19. If there is an effective medicine or therapy against Covid-19, which is the case, then vaccines become unnecessary.

Numerous experimental mRNA materials, which technically are genetic therapy and not true vaccines, have nevertheless been rushed into production at "warp speed", and without adequate animal or human testing. A panicked and misled public today lines up for them, eager for the hoped-for "heaven" of unlocked and mask-free living. It was an empty promise, as the vaccinated public is now learning. They are told to continue masking, lockdowns and social isolation. And clever media propaganda now blames the "unvaccinated" as if they are toxic, germ-infested unclean people, the same ugly propaganda the Nazis used to demonize Jews, Gypsies, and other "untermenschen". We now hear of "vaccine passports" that will segregate unvaccinated people into second-class citizenship, with a loss of rights to travel and work, and with bans for entry into entire fear-possessed slave-nations, as well as into concerts, sports events, and elsewhere. All that's needed are swastika arm-bands for the "clean übermensch" vaccinated, and a Star of David badge for the unvaccinated. History tells us what proceeds thereon.

    With all such incredible things going on, it is no wonder that large percentages of people are refusing to take the risky mRNA "vaccinations", ignoring the massive propaganda campaign aimed at them, and rebelling against the entire structure of the growing Medical Police State.

Changing Definitions of a Disease Case

    Another important factor is how the older medical determinations of a "disease case" have been far more loosely defined today, to the point of serious and deadly error. For example, a sick person once was said to have a *case* of a disease, such as tuberculosis, when they had the actual and clearly identifiable symptoms of that disease. For TB it is persisting cough often with blood, chest pain, loss of appetite and weight, fatigue, fever, chills, night sweats, and also with the TB bacterium present at high levels in their body fluids. That is the "old fashioned" fact-driven case-diagnosis and epidemiology. By contrast, today a "case" of Covid-19 is "diagnosed" merely by use of an error-prone PCR or antigen biochemical testing method. One does not need to have symptoms of Covid-19 to be identified as a "confirmed case" where it is *assumed, without scientific evidence or justification,* that by a positive biochemical test, you have living infectious Covid-19 virus within your system. And from there the unproven claim is made that such a "case" person is at risk of Covid-19 sickness, and of infecting other people. Taken with claims of new viral mutations, "official truth" science, medicine and politics pushes for ever-longer lockdowns and forced masking, in a never-ending spiral of authoritarian and unconstitutional "edicts".

"Evidence-Based Medicine" Often Ignores the Evidence

Finally I should mention the general abandonment by modern virology of Koch's Postulates for identification of a pathogen causing a specific disease. Those postulates are similar to rules of evidence used by police when trying to solve a murder – such as fingerprinting, ballistics testing, and eye witness reports. For microbial diseases, they include:

1) The microorganism must be present in every case of the disease.

2) The microorganism must be isolated from the host with the disease and grown in pure culture.

3) The specific disease must be reproduced when a pure culture of the microorganism is inoculated into a healthy susceptible host.

4) The microorganism must be recoverable from the experimentally infected host, but not from the uninfected.

Item number 2 above is a sticking point for claimed viral disorders, such as HIV or the Hepatitis C virus, for which environmental or lifestyle factors within narrow high-risk groups play the major role in immune-system stress and sickness. Space does not permit a full discussion of Koch's Postulates and its growing abandonment, but it seems necessary to point out how the corona viruses have not been isolated in pure cultures by which their pathogenicity on lab animals could be identified in conditions free of other factors. And that weakens the large claims of the new "warp speed" vaccines supposedly based upon such viruses. By side-stepping Koch's Postulates, modern medicine is frequently at odds with epidemiology, biology and other science disciplines, in determining the true causes of diseases, and their most effective treatments.

Modern medicine has also become increasingly centralized and government regulated, rarely to the betterment of the public health or the honest physician. Growing governmental "command and control" measures, as found in the UK National Health Service, the USA Medicare, and later "Obama-care", increasingly obliterated the independent physician and small clinic. Also the new methods of "test-kit" medicine transferred much of traditional diagnosis from the physician to the laboratory technician, whose presumed skills and laboratory machinery conceal an abundance of unstated or frequently wrong assumptions. It is not merely how AIDS and Covid-19 were/are "diagnosed" by faulty PCR tests. False diagnoses can be deadly when a white-coated authority figure basically points a "finger of doom" at sick or healthy people, potentially sending them into an emotional panic death-spiral. The claimed "viral causation" of both AIDS and Covid-19 have never been proven, and as this book shows, there is much which weighs against any clear or unchallenged corona-virus cause for the claimed "unique Covid-19 disease".

This "testing mania" is also a big problem in the widely used but inaccurate PSA test for prostate cancer, which results in a lot of unnecessary surgery, sometimes leaving older men incontinent and in a worse condition than before the surgery. Genetic tests for female breast cancer susceptibility are similarly questionable, rooted in unproven genetic calculus, and also leading to unnecessary surgical mutilations where no demonstrable symptoms of cancer are present, just a "test".

Entire books have been written on these subjects, on the over-reach and deadly nature of certain branches of modern medicine. Today's claims of viral or genetic causation of diseases often become the abandoned theories of tomorrow, for what are later proven to be environmental, dietary or emotion-driven maladies. Genetics and biochemistry have their place, and successes, but far too many failures.

I will end this section by sharing a Covid-19 anecdote of a "death by hospital" which happened to a local friend's father. The elderly man, about 80 years old, developed a cough and fever, typical of influenza. In a panic about Covid-19, his wife rushed him by car to the hospital emergency room. Upon arrival, the medical staff came out in full hazmat gear, and put him on a stretcher and took him inside, while the wife went and parked the car. A few minutes later, after returning to the emergency room, her husband was not to be seen. She asked around, and the attending young physician told her the man had been moved to an isolation ward. She was told she could not see him anymore, even though he was alert and lucid just a few minutes earlier, and although she had been in intimate contact with her husband as his cough and fever developed. Confused, she went home and called her relatives, who came with her to the hospital the next day. They confronted the head doctor, demanding to see the old man, but were again refused. "He has Covid-19 and is now on a ventilator, and cannot be visited or moved anymore." They were not allowed to even see him through a window-glass, and the old man was given a nearly hopeless diagnosis. The family asked the doctor to try high-dose vitamin C therapy, which elicited only a nasty curled-lip denunciation of that idea by the ignorant doctor. The family was cowed and beaten down by the arrogant, authoritarian doctor and hospital staff, and in my opinion they should have contacted a lawyer with the disposition of a junk-yard dog, to threaten the hospital and doctor with a lawsuit unless their concerns were addressed. In any case, the old man died a few days later, not given any kind of helpful medicine. He was instead left to die alone, drugged into semi-conscious paralysis by the hospital staff to keep him from trying to disconnect from the ventilator. What a Hellish way to die!

Now, this is not an isolated example, I've heard similar accounts from other people and nurses, along with more positive reports where elderly people with serious influenza symptoms did not go to the hospital and recovered by using the remedies mentioned above. If I was sick with a Covid-19 "diagnosis" or "test", I would NEVER go to hospitals, *especially if I had symptoms mirroring an ordinary cold or flu.* If a deep-lung problem existed, standard antibiotics might be necessary, but *only* on an out-patient basis. Grandma's chicken soup with plenty of garlic, high dose vitamin C (5-20 grams daily as calcium ascorbate powder in water or juice), vitamin D (10,000 or more for some days), zinc supplements and other natural remedies would provide a much better chance of recovery. A prescription for hydroxychloroquine or ivermectin would also be sought, and I would also use the "heretical" orgone energy blanket for bioenergy boosting.[81] Of course, a supportive and loving family, a healthy lifestyle, good water, clean air, nutrition, vitamins, minerals and preventive steps *before getting sick* is the best solution of all.

2021: Covid Madness and Vaccine Terrorism

The above material lays out the evidence, that the current theory about Covid-19 disease being caused by a specific identified SARS-CoV-2 virus is seriously flawed and lacks scientifically-defendable proof on every major point. The theories of pathogenic, infectious virology fail to explain why the "cases" do not predict actual deaths, of who lives or dies, or even who gets sick or stays healthy. The PCR or antigen testing, or even more subjective clinical diagnoses, have all proven inadequate to determine future morbidity or mortality. *These failures are hallmarks of a bad and inaccurate theory.* A good theory predicts how things will proceed, what is cause and what is effect, and allows for reliable measures and new findings to emerge supporting its original basic assumptions. None of this is true for the theory of claimed viral-caused Covid-19 disease.

Covid-19 disease has numerous similarities to many other diseases and conditions – the so-called "comorbidities" which are actually killing people (4 deadly comorbidities on average for each "Covid-19" death). These facts alone suggest Covid-19 is an unnecessary and erroneous construct of modern pharmaceutical-driven allopathic medicine.

The issues of profiteering by medical and pharmaceutical interests have not been explicitly discussed in this work, given our focus upon basic issues of scientific proofs. But it is a subject deserving of serious investigation. How is it that so many of the "health experts" who ascend to top positions in government and mainstream media predictably parrot the same kind of fear-mongering hysteria, and always dismiss or even slander the larger number of honest physicians and scientists who disagree? Are the government-selected doctors now our new Gods? Does the doctor's White Coat now replace the old Black Robe of the religious priesthood? Likewise, the role of mainstream media and medical-health societies and bureaucracies, in their push to silence dissent in medicine and science, and also to erase American freedoms in favor of a growing Medical Police State, deserves immediate public skepticism and disobedience, as well as eventual criminal prosecutions at every level of government. As per the important quote by Benjamin Rush on page 3 of this book.

This behavior of the top power structure has led to an erosion of freedoms not seen at any time except during the Revolutionary War, and later Civil War, and then being only temporary. Today, June of 2021, there is finally an accelerating public skepticism for the overall Covid-19 litany, and this is healthy. But it has come at a high price for the national awakening. Over 300,000 deaths in 2020. An additional approximate 200,000+ claimed deaths have so far occurred as of June 2021. All such numbers are suspect, however, given the unreliable PCR-claimed case-death non-causality as already discussed. But the government-dictated lockdowns and hysteria, which I consider to be *the real causes of such deaths in 2020*, have continued more or less. In 2021, even as the numbers of cases and deaths have declined dramatically in the USA, a new deadly "comorbidity" has appeared, in the form of *reckless experimental gene-therapy "vaccines".*

According to VAERS (Vaccine Adverse Event Reporting System), maintained by the CDC, a total of 4170 people of all ages had died from vaccine sickness as of 24 May and 14,506 deaths as of 3 September, 2021.[82] That is far more deaths than from the 911 terror attacks – and yet, look at the stark differences in how these two numbers of dead people are treated by governments, media, medical doctors and the general public? I personally reviewed the VAERS data to obtain that number, as well as the other data tables and graphs presented below. Comparisons to vaccine deaths in prior years illuminates this outrageous situation.

Influenza vaccines are voluntarily accepted by around 165 million Americans each year. While their efficacy is nevertheless in question, the number of deaths from them remains quite low, at around 200 persons per year. Even when adding up all vaccine death numbers, they have been dramatically low by comparison to what is happening now, in 2021, with the Covid-19 "vaccines". Table L presents the actual numbers.

Figures 15 and 16 graphically depict these same Table L death data, as well as the "Other Adverse Reactions" data as extracted from the VAERS data posted to the CDC website on 24 May 2021.[82]

Given the massive "warp speed" numbers of Covid-19 vaccines being administered, the majority of 2021 vaccine deaths and adverse reactions are from the Covid-19 vaccines. For example, from late December 2020 to 24 March 2021, around half of all Americans, around 160 million people, have received one or more of the various Covid-19 shots, as well as other vaccinations. If the Covid-19 vaccinations were as mild as the flu shots, then we should expect the numbers of Covid-19 vaccine deaths to be about the same as flu vaccines over the last several years. This is not the case. Flu vaccines and all other vaccines for the years prior to 2021 ranged from a low of 77 deaths in 1990, to a high of 223 in 1995. The average over the 32 year period from 1990 through 2020 is 158 deaths. Consequently we cannot rationally compare the influenza or any other vaccines with those being administered for claimed Covid-19. The evidence appears solid, that the Covid-19 vaccines (or experimental

Table L: Deaths From All Vaccines, by Year [82]			
Year	Deaths	Year	Deaths
1990	77	2007	162
1991	160	2008	182
1992	218	2009	191
1993	219	2010	161
1994	223	2011	173
1995	140	2012	166
1996	124	2013	129
1997	134	2014	131
1998	132	2015	149
1999	144	2016	177
2000	141	2017	121
2001	174	2018	164
2002	135	2019	183
2003	199	2020	166
2004	162	2021- 24 May	4,170
2005	131	2021- 3 Sep.	14,506
2006	123	2021- Full Year	~20,000?

Figure 15 Annual Vaccine Deaths (VAERS)[82]

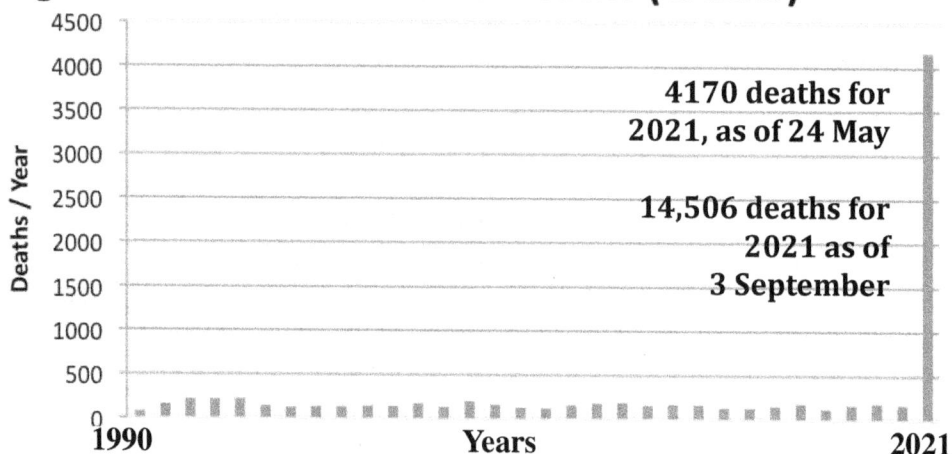

gene therapy shots) must be far more deadly than prior vaccines, given the dramatically higher numbers of toxic human reactions to them. This would be due to their highly experimental nature, and lack of adequate animal or human testing before they were rushed and unleashed upon an unsuspecting and panicked public.

As of early September of 2021, the VAERS death-count from the Covid-19 vaccines has reached 14,506, while the Adverse Reactions soaring to 675,593. The vaccine death numbers may be much higher, given how there is no medical mandate to report adverse reactions to VAERS, which is an entirely voluntary program. So the actual numbers of unreported Covid-19 vaccine deaths could raise the death toll by an order of magnitude (10 times!), and those extra death numbers would just blend in with the background of "all cause" death statistics.

It is a national disgrace that no "high-up" people promoting this massive and unnecessary vaccine campaign – replete with overtones of Nazi-like totalitarian "vaccine passports" – is bothered by these vaccine death and serious injury numbers, just as they ignored the probable cause of the even larger number of deaths, in the hundreds of thousands, due to government-dictated lockdowns, despair and economic ruin!

Whatever the actual number of vaccine deaths may be, at minimum we are witnessing far more vaccine deaths in 2021 than the cumulative total of vaccine deaths from 1994 through 2020. Should that trend continue until the end of 2021, the vaccine deaths would rise to around 20,000. No wonder why so many educated people are refusing to "take the shot".

Figure 16 Other Annual Adverse Vaccine Reactions (mild to severe, VAERS)[82]

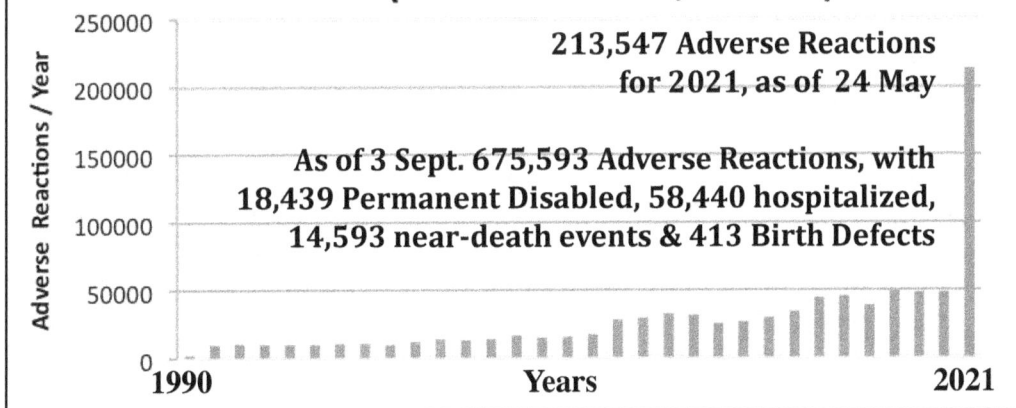

213,547 Adverse Reactions for 2021, as of 24 May

As of 3 Sept. 675,593 Adverse Reactions, with 18,439 Permanent Disabled, 58,440 hospitalized, 14,593 near-death events & 413 Birth Defects

Adverse Reactions / Year

250000, 200000, 150000, 100000, 50000, 0

1990   Years   2021

The European death-data is worse. As of 17 April 2021, the EU recorded 330,218 Covid vaccine injury reports (from all four available COVID vaccines), including 7,766 deaths. By June, EU vaccine deaths went over 15,000. By September, the EU deaths probably exceeded 20,000. By another comparison, in 1976 around 45 million Americans took the Swine Flu vaccine, which was halted and banned after *only 54 deaths*.

Meanwhile "adverse events" of mild to severe illness following Covid-19 shots are commonplace across the USA, including for children as a form of "government-mandated child abuse". As of May 24, VAERS received over 900 reports among 12- to 17-year old Covid-vaccinated youth who developed heart inflammation disorders like myocarditis. And yet, according to my Tables I and J, young people below the age of 24 have essentially a ZERO statistical risk of death from Covid-19 as compared to the non-Covid "all cause" deaths which afflict those same younger groups. Young people die sometimes, but overwhelmingly from accidents, suicides or identified comorbidities, not from Covid-19 – except for more than a year we have the added stressor of isolation misery and health-injury inflicted upon them by the lockdowns and forced masking. They do not need added pain and injury from unnecessary "Covid vaccines". Nor does anyone else.

Beyond the minimal 14,506 deaths and 675.593 serious adverse events identified by VAERS for just the first 9 months of 2021, there is growing evidence that people who get the vaccines are at risk to subsequently "test positive" on the inaccurate PCR tests, the so-called "breakthrough cases" previously mentioned, leading to public health confusions with additional alarm. Such cases have risen dramatically indicating the vaccines don't work, and that the "variant" breakthroughs are in fact nothing but the deadly side-effects of the mRNA experimental shots. The medical profession remains in denial, however, and largely goes along with the CDC's gargantuan lie, lowering the cycle threshold of PCR machines for vaccinated people to better erase the "breakthroughs", insuring more of the unvaccinated refuseniks will "test positive" by comparison, even if perfectly healthy and having already achieved natural herd immunity. This one factor alone exposes the criminal nature of the CDC's methodology, like putting a gun to the heads of the general public, to coerce them into false beliefs that the experimental mRNA Covid vaccines are "safe" and the unvaccinated are "dirty infectious people, a risk to everyone else".[42]

Figure 17 displays the current Covid-19 cases and deaths in graphic form. I've already discussed in detail the most rational causes for the peaks in cases (not reflected in deaths, however) at points A, B and C. On a cursory review, it would appear the most recent fourth peak in the Covid-19 "cases" from mid February to late May 2021, is the result of the widespread experimental Covid-19 shots themselves. The dotted black line provides an hypothetical, but probable incidence curve had the mRNA experimental injections *not been granted "Experimental Use Authorization" status by the FDA.*

From all the above, it is not surprising that the number of PCR-identified "Covid cases" and also deaths have increased somewhat shortly after the mRNA Covid-19 shots were introduced. The best presentation on that comes from a privately developed YouTube video (not yet censored) using the same Our World in Data website graphics for each nation, identifying the late December 2020 or early 2021 time when the vaccines were introduced.[83] In just about every nation, the death rates go up shortly afterwards, not down. Few or none of those deaths are being attributed to the vaccines, even while the correlation to their introduction is reasonable. While the death numbers presented in that reference are not so high as compared to the overall "Covid-19" PCR-claimed deaths (the comorbidities), it is further evidence that these rushed and coerced experimental mRNA injection programs are not having the intended effects, as increasing numbers of people are refusing to participate.

These additional and unnecessary numbers of dead and sickened people, some with life-long injuries, are outrageous. The silence of mainstream medicine and media about it is a continuation of similar silence during the whole of 2020, in the face of massive contrary evidence to the

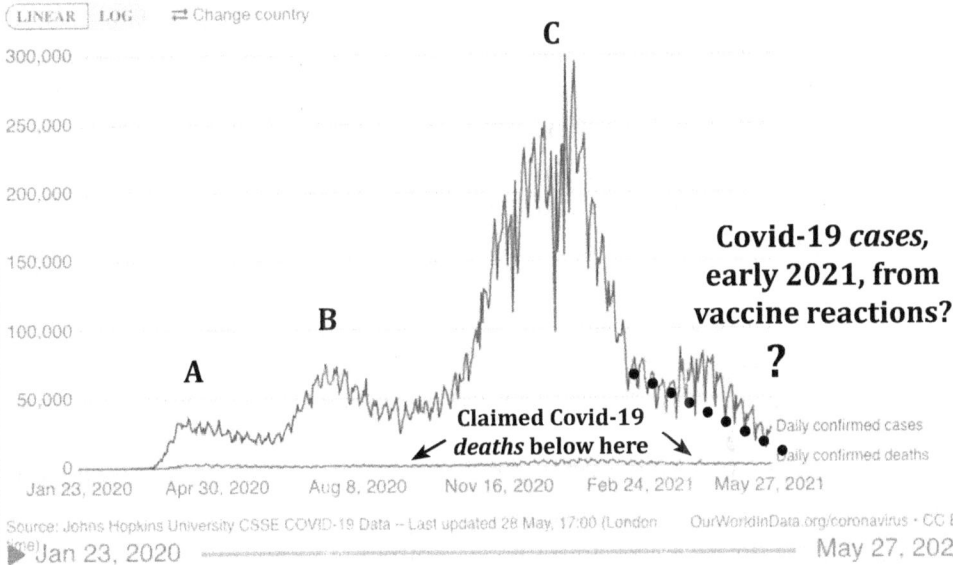

Daily confirmed COVID-19 cases and deaths, United States

Our World in Data

The confirmed counts shown here are lower than the total counts. The main reason for this is limited testing and challenges in the attribution of the cause of death.

LINEAR   LOG   ⇄ Change country

Covid-19 *cases,* early 2021, from vaccine reactions?

?

Claimed Covid-19 *deaths* below here

Daily confirmed cases
Daily confirmed deaths

A   B   C

300,000
250,000
200,000
150,000
100,000
50,000
0

Jan 23, 2020   Apr 30, 2020   Aug 8, 2020   Nov 16, 2020   Feb 24, 2021   May 27, 2021

Source: Johns Hopkins University CSSE COVID-19 Data – Last updated 28 May, 17:00 (London   OurWorldInData.org/coronavirus · CC BY

Jan 23, 2020   May 27, 2021

Figure 17. The Full American Pandemic Toll, from March 2020 through Late May 2021. Our World In Data.[15]

conventional lies and hooliganism of the national medical-media-political leadership, which led to lockdowns, masking, etc. It was and is a shameful discarding of the physician's oath, to *"First Do No Harm".* And now, many "health officials" just ignore these death data and serious injury reports, as if they were nothing, viewing the ordinary person with contempt, and their own efforts as some kind of righteous *Holy War.* On the public side of this pathological equation, we see narcissistic displays of overly-enthusiastic citizen obedience, bordering on self-asserted "heroism", to "take the shot" and suffer its possible bad effects "with a stiff upper lip", as if one was "fighting on" in the same Holy War. Comparisons are also seen to a Covid religious fervor, with self-righteous attitudes of superiority. Fighting Covid is like "fighting the Devil", and "taking the shot" a cleansing by Holy Water. And if you dare question the heroic saints of Covid, such as St. Fauci, or St. Gates, then you are greeted with curled-lip hatred and curses, including banishment from workplaces, social groups and even families. The same emotional dynamic once led to real Holy Wars.

And yet, just as with religious or political extremism, there is a price the "superior" vaccinated individuals and society will pay, that cannot be avoided. While that VAERS number of 14,506 dead, or the extrapolated prediction of 20,000+ vaccine-caused deaths by the end of 2021 are relatively small by comparison to the hundreds of thousands of extra deaths from claimed "Covid-19" (the comorbidities), there are troubling expert opinions – from *real experts* – warning of declining health among the Covid vaccinated over the next few years. For example, there may be possible increased degenerative and auto-immune reactions yet to come. Or, the vaccinated may suffer from alterations in their DNA, with possible sterility, and also that the vaccinated are the source of the new "variants", being dangerous to others. Whatever the truth or error in those concerns, it is very clear that the mainstream advocates of this current coercive or forced vaccination program have their own basket of ugly junk-science and Big Lies to spread.

Remember again, *there is no evidence whatsoever to the claim that "herd immunity can only be achieved by widespread vaccinations",* as once famously stated by the top American "High Priest of Vaccines", Anthony Fauci, and other medical Grand Inquisitors. That statement was conjured up as a means to further down-play the use of inexpensive medicines such as hydroxychloroquine, ivermectin, vitamins C, D and zinc supplements (previously discussed) to combat "Covid-19", which in most cases expresses itself with mild cold or flu symptoms. (Or it is the cold or flu.) Had those medicines been used widely at the start of the Covid -19 panic, death numbers would have dropped dramatically, mirroring ordinary influenza, and the mRNA shots would not have been "necessary".

There are millions of people who, if PCR-virus theory is to be believed, were already exposed to SARS-CoV-2, tested positive, became slighly ill with flu symptoms or remained asymptomatic, or had only mild symptoms. By classical biology and epidemiology, that very large group of people is already immune and does not need any vaccinations. And yet, the CDC pushes vaccination of everyone, even if their natural immunity is stronger than claimed "vaccine immunity". Then there are millions of younger people who by their natural healthy condition, are at nearly zero risk. But those facts fall upon deaf ears of mainsream medicine, even if they are formulated from within the Covid-19 disease paradigm, and use the CDC's own data as I do in this book.

Again, nowhere in the USA, during any time of this claimed virus-caused Covid-19 pandemic has anyone been forced to haul dead bodies out to mass-graves, nor to bury their neighbors. Nothing like it. And just from that direct observation, which nobody can counter with any factual examples, we must ask if this whole deadly drama of 2020 and now 2021 is merely a Saint-Vitus Dance of public psychoses and hysteria, a living-out of various Hollywood fiction movies about deadly plagues that wipe out entire populations, and the heroic white-coated doctors and experts who *save the world* (by shooting vaccine refusers, in one notable film). But that is an unreality, a fiction. History tells us, such an alignment of medical/scientific "experts" working in collusion with Big Government, Big Media, and Big Industry are more likely to be the most dangerous constellation of power one should be worried about. Think Lysenkoism. Think Hitlerism. Think Stalinism. Pick your historical period, and you'll see it. We see it growing now, today, with Covid-19, and also obvious is that the power-drunk elements don't want it to end, and so they continually raise the bar, about some new "variant", some new excuse to "extend the lockdowns, just another month or two". We are now a full year beyond the original shabby excuses for this *Covid Terrorism*.

By the numbers, it appears that only around 50% of the American public will have taken the vaccines, with increasing numbers of people expressing skepticism about their safety, and hence refusing them. Organized bullies in Big Government and Big Medicine are of course alarmed at the "refuseniks" and try to coerce or punish people, with vaccine propaganda and Nazi-like "passports". They are pushing new edicts to vaccinate all children before schools can reopen, which is patently junk science and official deadly child abuse. Again, one can see in my Tables I and J, the numbers of which were obtained directly from the CDC, where the percentages of young people dying of what they call Covid-19 is fleetingly small, at a percentage nearly identical to the general deaths of those younger age groups from "all causes". Over the entire year of 2020, there were ZERO excess deaths from Covid-19 in the under 24-years age groups, by comparison to those in the "all cause" groups. And the deaths of the older groups got classified as "Covid-19" only by error-prone PCR, antigen, and subjective clinical determinations. There is a form of academic-medical "group-think" at work, where the "experts" simply cannot think outside of their self-created box.

Beyond these lingering challenges in 2021, and my conclusions as given in the prior sections, I continue to feel suspicious about the CDC's last-minute data-dumps – the 269,249 new all-cause deaths reported in the last week of 2020, and the added boost of 87,000 into the Covid-19 death numbers in early 2021. There may be innocence to some part of the number-boosts, as with updated death counts during the last week of December 2020 and in January 2021. However, *the way in which it was done suggested a deliberate effort to spread more public panic and hysteria.*

Conclusions and Recommendations

The analysis and points made in this book focus upon the USA Covid data and situation over 2020 and the first half of 2021. They are also valid, by extrapolation, for all other nations trapped in the Covid nightmare.

* The medical symptoms of Covid-19 considerably overlap with those of ordinary upper and lower respiratory illness, such as influenza or pneumonia, further suggesting claimed Covid-19 infections are those other known respiratory diseases and disorders.

* Claimed Covid-19 deaths are 81% confined to elderly people over 65 years old, and 93% over 55. *The vast majority of people perishing in this elderly group had an average of 4 pre-existing deadly comorbidities, already approaching an "end of life" phase.* Only around 5% of Covid-19 deaths had no comorbidities.

* Winter seasonality of Covid-19 deaths affirms a relationship to standard influenza and pneumonia, as well as to other maladies that are exacerbated by cold wet weather. Possible misdiagnosis of those known conditions and diseases as Covid-19 is strongly indicated by this one factor alone. Deaths by pneumonia, influenza and other comorbidities are in many cases being deliberately mixed up with Covid-19 deaths in government health agencies, further indicating inaccuracies in Covid-19 diagnoses. Covid-19 deaths are thereby *magnified*, with a disappearance of usual wintertime deaths from influenza and flu-like conditions.

* Electron microscopy does not reveal any clearly specific or pure-culture image of SARS-CoV-2, the virus blamed for Covid-19, and cannot conclusively distinguish it from other corona viruses. Similarly, diagnostic x-rays show typical "ground glass" or opacities in the lung for numerous lung disorders, and not merely for the claimed Covid-19.

* While Covid-19 tests and cases have soared, neither are correlated to, nor predict the much smaller number of Covid-19 deaths. Covid-19 death/case ratios, and death/test ratios, were at a moderately higher level initially in 2020 when PCR/Antigen tests were isolated to those in hospitals with high levels of comorbidity. Those ratios declined rapidly when laboratory tests were applied to the larger population of healthy and asymptomatic people outside of hospitals.

* PCR testing for Covid-19 is highly error-prone due to the intrinsic high sensitivity of that method, especially when the numbers of cycles on PCR-testing machinery are set too high. PCR test methods react to many things, including dead virus, non-living viral DNA/RNA fragments, and antibodies created by healthy people to all kinds of other corona viruses, and who otherwise are not at risk of the disease, or of spreading it. *If one needs to use PCR to detect a virus, then there cannot be enough of it in the body by which biochemical significance could be achieved. This also indicates such a claimed virus is not replicating itself, nor is it infectious.*

* Inaccurate PCR laboratory tests, rather than a living infectious deadly virus SARS-CoV-2, *created the "Covid-19 cases"*. From such test result inaccuracies, one cannot say who will or will not get sick, or who will or will not die, aside from possible induced psychosomatic alarm and social upset due to an hysterically presumed "Covid-19 Death Sentence". As such, the PCR tests are shown to have *No Predictive Value*, which is *the hallmark of a bad scientific theory.* The entire theoretical basis of a new and unique "Covid-19 pandemic" thereby appears as only a virological illusion, an artificial diagnostic and theoretical construct, irrespective of how many "excess" elderly people were or are dying.

* Covid-19 cases have soared only due to tens of millions of unnecessary and faulty PCR/Antigen tests being made on the generally healthy and asymptomatic population. *Herd Immunity,* as an expression of widespread resistance to all flu-like infections, including seasonal Covid-19 (whatever that truly is) was achieved over summer of 2020.

* The age-group percentages of Covid-19 deaths are not significantly different from those perishing in the same age group from all other causes. The "excess deaths" calculation reported here indicates no more than 5400 elderly people died from claimed Covid-19 by comparison to the same age groups dying from all other causes. As noted above, this further undermines the claims of an infectious deadly viral pandemic.

* Those older folk who were sick and dying should have been diagnosed and treated according to pre-Covid-19 symptomology, by the so-called "comorbidities", which are the real causes of their illness. Effective and inexpensive medicines already existed for such treatment outside of hospitals. These medicines were politically suppressed by the "health" bureaucracies, however, while expensive and marginally effective pharmaceuticals were promoted to the public, along with risky vaccines.

* Hospitals were paid extra sums by government health agencies to *lie on death certificates and reclassify the many comorbidity deaths as "Covid-19", to jack up the numbers.*

* Ending of lockdowns, forced masking and isolation have not led to an increase in cases or deaths, just the opposite. Lockdown "slave states" have suffered the most, while "free states" thrived. The "New Normal" of lockdowns, etc., is *a form of state-sanctioned iatrogenic murder.*

* The new Covid-19 vaccines are publicly misrepresented and are actually genetic therapy injections, using messenger-RNA (mRNA) to transplant new genetic material into the test subject. These vaccines were rushed into production without significant animal or human testing, which is now being done on a mass scale on human populations without informed consent. The vaccines required "emergency approvals" from the FDA. They do not appear effective as demonstrated by the many "vaccine breakthrough cases" where people confusedly test positive after receiving the injections. Efforts are underway to cover-up this serious problem undermining the vaccine propaganda, by lowering the cycle-threshold sensitivity of PCR-test equipment for the vaccinated, so fewer "breakthrough cases" will be detected. This is not being done for the unvaccinated, however, exposing yet another major CDC deception.

* From January through early September of 2021, according to the VAERS data, some 14,506 people have died from the Covid-19 vaccines. Extrapolated to the year's end, that would result in around 20,000 vaccine deaths. *That is far greater than all the cumulative deaths recorded from all other vaccines since the VAERS reporting system was initiated in 1990.* Prior vaccine programs were ended after as few as 50 or 60 persons had died. Those supporting this deadly pro-vaccine hysteria also push for *Nazi-like "vaccine passports" and other inhuman segregationist slave-state policies.* These policies reveal an arrogant, deadly attitude, fully in violation of the Nuremberg Code drafted after WW2, the US Constitution's limitations on government power, and also the ancient physician's oath, to ***"First Do No Harm"!***

* Many ignorant or compromised physicians, mainstream media stars and internet billionaires have colluded with the worst of power-drunk government bureaucrats and pharmaceutical profiteers, to censor and criminalize scientific and medical dissent. Citizen protests have also been brutally suppressed, with an acquiescing silent nod of approval from the scientific, medical, media and political mainstream.

* The disruptions of normal life due to Covid-19 hysteria, lockdowns and forced masking have their own deadly pathology. A large number of people died from pre-existing comorbidities amplified psychosomatically by lockdowns, forced masking, social isolation and economic ruin, all of which created immense fear, panic, and despair. *Those factors have been deliberately and systematically ignored by the "experts in power" throughout this claimed viral pandemic.* Only a few private working groups in a few universities, and a few individual scientists or physicians working alone, have investigated this situation, affirming a new and deadly iatrogenic disaster.

* By my own rough estimates, *252,750 extra people died* in the severely locked-down states, who did not die in the low- or no-lockdown states. (See my Table C on page 42.) *An additional 416,820 people died* as extra deaths due to the various effects of severe lockdowns, forced masking, isolation-distancing, economic ruin and deaths by despair. (See my Table F on page 50). These death numbers get little or no interest or attention from the big-shots of medicine, media, or politics. They are the lost souls, thrown overboard by a misinformed society, discussed only by small numbers of censored and erased scholars who know the facts and review the data accordingly.

* The *mass psychology of the Covid-19 hysteria* is granting social permissions for ordinary people to become "volunteers" in a new medical Holy War, acting as social spies and censors of their own family, friends, neighbors and fellow citizens. "See Something, Say Something" was a slogan once formulated regarding terrorists planting bombs. Today it has morphed into calling the police if someone is hosting a party, or seen walking around without a face-mask, or not adequately "distancing". Nasty and hateful attitudes buried in the human character are today allowed free expression within the context of Covid-19. As Orwell wrote in his fictional novel *1984*, we have a powerful new "Ministry of Truth" growing within our social institutions. Our WHO, CDC, NIH, FDA and other large and small government institutions are, with collaboration of mainstream media, "health" bureaucracies, internet billionaires and reckless private foundations (WEF, GF, RF, etc.), actively re-defining important words, erasing contrary science and data, and censoring and slandering dissenting voices. By such measures, psychopaths have gained controls within our government and institutions, and seek to deliberately wreak havoc upon an unsuspecting but also often Big-Brother-Loving population. This is expressed on the social scene as hatred of those who dissent, object, or refuse to "go along to get along". It is an *Emotional Plague* that can infect entire nations and take them down into self-imposed disasters, as described by the psychiatrist Wilhelm Reich who wrote penetrating analyses of the social catastrophes in Nazi Germany and Communist Russia. For doing so, he also was slandered, censored, *had his books burned by the FDA, and died in prison in 1957* for his breakthrough discoveries. What we see today on the social scene is moving in a similar direction.

There is a terrible stench of "official truth" Orwellian deception in every facet of this claimed Covid-19 pandemic. *The manner in which so many dissenting voices of both professionals and laypeople, challenging the "official truth" of Covid-19, are rudely or brutally censored and erased from mainstream media reports, and from internet social media, is exactly what one anticipates during a widespread political/medical cover-up.* It also makes understandable the fearful paralysis, as well as the outrage seen among different sectors of the general public, against this *Official Covid Terrorism* within a growing *Medical Police State.*

The various issues raised in this analysis lead to staggering new open questions, and to a completely different set of critical conclusions about Covid-19: Incongruent case-death data, seasonal variations, similarities and overlaps in clinical diagnoses between what is influenza or pneumonia versus what is Covid-19 disease, electron micrograph puzzles, PCR/Antigen testing inaccuracies, trends in population and deaths, lockdowns and *Death by Despair*, and few or nobody in "official science" using the straightforward single-year method I report to determine "excess deaths". Abundant evidence points to a *pandemic of error, terror and hysteria.*

This current "pandemic" is one of misdiagnoses, of overlapping categories of illness, of fraudulent book-keeping, and of inaccurate PCR and antigen tests, where seasonal wintertime influenza, pneumonia, colds and various respiratory disorders are being misidentified as Covid-19. Beyond the criticisms of conventional Covid-19 thinking, I am forced to raise open questions on the real reasons for the many extra deaths over 2020.

Are these numerous additional deaths the consequence of totalitarian lockdowns, exacerbated pre-existing comorbidities, of added anxiety, hysteria and panic, and economic ruin driving Death by Despair to ever higher numbers? And is it not so, that once so simplistically "diagnosed" as Covid-19, those who rush to hospitals for help rarely receive the inexpensive, clinically proven remedies? Under mainstream conventional care, such hospitalized patients almost always are given expensive toxic drugs, put on often-deadly ventilators, subjected to a hellish set of abusive treatments in profiteering hospitals staffed by nurses and physicians with a "Holy War" mentality. And what does "Holy War mentality" mean exactly? It means the physicians and hospital staff are so busy "fighting in the trenches" against what they conceive to be a deadly enemy virus-plague, that they don't wish to be distracted, and don't have time or patience for anyone who dares to question their group-think Covid Religion. This is so, even when so much of their own advocacy and ministrations wreak havoc upon human society and biology, worsening real symptoms and making despair and death more probable. And from that ideological rigidity, they can easily ignore the critics, even within their own profession, ignore also the massive totalitarian political shift in our social structure, ignore the plight and blight created by government-planned and anti-Constitutional ordering of economic ruin. Do they view such social destruction and deaths as "necessary sacrifices during a medical anti-virus Holy War?"

I regrettably conclude that this is, indeed, what has happened over our *Lost Year* of 2020, which now expands into 2021.

The usual scientific approach of epidemiology was abandoned over this Covid-19 epoch. Covid-19 was *politically weaponized*, ushering in violent intolerance within government, media and medicine for those asking certain "wrong" questions. As noted, *there are no official scientific or medical working groups in the entire USA, not in Federal, State, County or City governments, who are both funded and dedicated to the full-time task of estimating deaths directly due to the hysterical Covid-19 lockdowns!* Neither does the WHO or UN have anyone studying this issue, even as numerous political-class dictators bark out orders for even more stringent and never-ending lockdowns and masking. They just assume the lockdowns, masking and economic ruin is "good medicine!" What deadly arrogance!

There are a few private individuals, like myself, and private groups of scientists and physicians working without significant funding, in their spare time, to document these factors. I have cited most of them. However, every one of them is under severe attack and personal slanders from Big Government, Big Medicine, Big Science, Big Pharma, and Big Internet. Their statements and personal testimonies are being censored, deleted from YouTube, Facebook, Twitter, Instagram, and other social media. Even their private websites get deleted by the vast networks of web servers owned and run by communist-minded Amazon corporation, which has also been deleting scientific books from its offerings that dare to dissent from conventional Covid theory or the necessity of vaccinations. These courageous individuals and smaller groups do their work without the usual benefits of funding or social tolerance that greets the mainstream pro-Covid propagandists at every turn. They often pay a heavy personal price in deplatforming, legal attacks, firings and even criminal prosecutions for doing so. Some have committed suicide. Even reports on the censorship they suffer are censored, making the situation a near-total blackout of scientific opinion that goes against government policies and medical tyranny.

This author has shared peer-reviewed scientific research articles on internet, materials expressing skepticism against lockdowns or routine vaccinations as published in peer-reviewed mainstream medical or science journals. Those materials were quickly deleted from my Facebook and Twitter accounts, locking me out for several weeks, with threats to fully cancel my accounts if I did so again. I also must fear full censorship of this book, along with *additional* death-threats given the controversial nature of my other writings. Does anyone on the pro-Covid side have similar repercussions or worries, flowing from their deadly propaganda or actions? No. This by itself is revealing, of a major widespread deception and cover-up, suggesting the deadly mainstream knows exactly what they are doing. There is no ignorant innocence in their conduct.

Neither the WHO, CDC, NIH, FDA, nor any other official government agency has bothered to study the issue of deaths due to the lockdown hysteria. Therefore both they and the leaders of the medical profession, the health bureaucracies, the funding agencies, mass media and the politicians who advocated the lockdown disaster, who slandered and blocked effective medicines, *must bear the primary responsibility for all the claimed "Covid-19" deaths, and the mRNA "vaccine" deaths over 2020 and 2021.* They have too often behaved like tyrant psychopaths, malignantly negligent at best, dead-faced murderous at worst. A great *banality of evil.*

The actual real numbers of added deaths due to lockdowns and associated draconian dictates by power-drunk politicians may take years to be definitively identified. But it is increasingly apparent that *"Covid-19" is merely a substitute diagnosis for most of these deaths, being mis-classified in accordance with the error-prone Covid-19 theory and bogus PCR tests. And with a lot of medical profiteering and fraud in the mix.*

From all the above, and once again, I must conclude:

All of the "excess deaths" of 2020 are due to the media-driven public hysteria and panic over a claimed but minimally documented "super-virus". The high mortalities are resultant more directly from government-sanctioned economic disruption, forced unemployment, ensuing poverty and bankruptcies, isolated elderly succumbing to depression and despair, exacerbating multiple comorbidities, with added suicides, drug overdoses, homicides and other factors. The deaths are the product of the failed Covid-19 virus theory, which has resulted in the lockdowns and all the physical and emotional traumas which came as a consequence.

Recommendations:

1. There must be an immediate and total end to forced lockdowns, masking and inhuman distancing, with efforts to salvage the economic basis of normal healthy human life!

2. Intelligent protections of the elderly and those at high risk from all sorts of normal and known infectious diseases should continue, but without the strictly punitive, sadistic and cruel "protections" such as quarantine, forced masking and isolation removal from friends and families. Outdoor exposure to natural sunlight and fresh air is a life-enhancing and curative remedy all by itself, and must resume.

3. Proven but suppressed, slandered and inexpensive out-of-patent remedies for all kinds of respiratory diseases, such as high-dose vitamin C and D, zinc supplements, hydroxychloroquine, ivermectin and other inexpensive, out-of-patent medicines must be made fully available and recommended to the general public, to overcome the negative propaganda against them. The FDA must have its police powers revoked, to end their sending SWAT teams with machine-guns into private clinics!

4. There should also be a decisive end to medical-pharmaceutical propaganda advertisements in public media as was the case in prior decades. This quickly destroys the political-medical-media cartels.

5. The medical profession can no longer be trusted to hold a monopoly over the public health. The prosecution and slander of physicians who were critical of Covid, who choose to use the suppressed methods for treatment of their patients must also end. Those who have promoted this pandemic to the public, from the high perch of government offices, spreading falsehoods and hysteria, should also be prosecuted for Crimes Against Humanity, as in the Nuremberg Trials of Nazi leaders. This is especially necessary for those billionaires who personally profited from the lockdowns or deadly vaccines being peddled as a "cure", while simultaneously censoring books and private internet materials expressing contrary facts and opinions. *They have killed millions of people!*

6. The mRNA "vaccinations" must stop immediately. Programs of "vaccine passports" under any name must be banned, as a hallmark of fascist totalitarian ideology. Nazi and Communist tyrants do that. Free nations do not.

7. We must quickly return to the "old normal" not merely for reasons of public health, but also to protect and restore our Constitutional Republic and the liberties and freedoms stolen from the American people.

8. The analysis in this book has predominantly addressed the situation in the USA. However, by rational extension, the critical points and conclusions presented here are applicable for all world regions, as they go to the basic question of *scientifically-defendable causality*, or the lack thereof.

9. The public must be alerted to this serious situation of emotionally-plagued medical, media and academic misreporting, so as to halt and end their own neurotic self-destructive tendencies. The obedient acceptance of lockdowns, masking, anti-social distancing, especially under circumstances where NO potential for transmission of deadly viruses or bacteria exists (as when driving or walking outdoors, on the beach, in the forest, etc.) must be addressed as paranoid compulsive behavior. Likewise, the treating of friends and relatives like lepers, keeping children away from school or placing them into plastic cages as if they were laboratory rats, and many similar alarmingly Medieval and fractious conducts must end. None of it is rational, or necessary. It is irrational societal suicide, evidence of mass-psychological disorders, especially within the ranks of psychopathic, sadistic and power-drunk politicians, bureaucrats and medical officials, who seem happy to lead entire nations over a cliff.

10. *The issues surrounding Covid-19 and the related public health are not the exclusive province or domain of medical or scientific "experts", who in the largest measure have miserably failed the entire world.* National populations were and are put at high risk by ineffective and unscientific claims demanding never-ending obedience from the general public. How much longer can people blindly and irrationally accept orders from the Big State, to lock down, to wear masks, to anti-socially distance, to keep children out of school, to take risky gene-therapy injections and submit "proofs of papers" to social Nazis, to allow their businesses to shutter down into bankruptcy, and a hundred other outrages with *very deadly consequences?* Governors and police forces have been unconstitutionally empowered or self-appointed to enforce claimed "public health measures" of a highly unscientific and totalitarian nature, a thin tissue of cover for ending of human freedom, life and love.

We stand at a crossroads. Will the public and responsible individuals in medicine, media and government step forward and put a final end to the lockdown hysteria and all the terror and oppression that came with it? Or will the power-drunk deceivers continue to rule the world? However events develop, one thing is certain. This constellation of anti-freedom and anti-health sociopaths, the "top experts", media stars and despotic politicians, coupled with an alarmingly uncritical public obedience to their dictates, has already led the world into a gigantic disaster. Public exposure of their malignant incompetence with significant punishments are necessary, so as to prevent it from happening again.

THIS MUST END NOW!

Recommended Health-Freedom Organizations

For updated facts about Covid-19, for protecting your health during this crisis of mass hysteria, lockdowns, medical ignorance and arrogance, review these informative links:

America's Front-Line Doctors - www.americasfrontlinedoctors.com

Association of American Physicians and Surgeons - www.aapsonline.org

Children's Health Defense - childrenshealthdefense.org

Collateral Global - collateralglobal.org

CoviLeaks - covileaks.co.uk

Doctors for Covid Ethics - doctors4covidethics.medium.com

The Great Barrington (Doctors and Scientists) Declaration gbdeclaration.org

Green Med Info - greenmedinfo.com

Lockdown Resistance - endlockdowns.org

Lockdown Sceptics - lockdownsceptics.org

Reclaim the Net, Opposing Online Censorship - reclaimthenet.org

VAERS Analysis - vaersanalysis.info

World Doctors Alliance - worlddoctorsalliance.com

Contact these groups and find local chapters of like-minded citizens and professionals, for collective action against the Covid Despots.

Cited References

1. WHO Pandemic Preparedness, 2 Feb 2003. web.archive.org/web/20030202200410/http://www.who.int/csr/disease/influenza/pandemic/en/index.html

2. WHO Pandemic Preparedness, 3 Sep. 2009. web.archive.org/web/20090903155635/http://www.who.int/csr/disease/influenza/pandemic/en/

3. www.theepochtimes.com/cdc-investigating-heart-inflammation-in-covid-19-vaccinated-teens-young-adults_3826981.html   https://articles.mercola.com/sites/articles/archive/2021/05/22/tucker-carlson-covid-vaccine-deaths.aspx

4. *Scenarios for the Future of Technology and International Development,* Rockefeller Foundation, May 2010, p.18. archive.org/details/2010-scenarios-for-the-future-of-technology-and-international-development

5. Non-pharmaceutical public health measures for mitigating the risk and impact of epidemic and pandemic influenza. thefatemperor.com/wp-content/uploads/2020/11/WHO-Pandemic-Guidelines-2019.pdf (see page 3 in this weblink)

6. Corman V., et al.: "Detection of 2019 novel coronavirus (2019-nCoV) by real-time RT-PCR" (Eurosurveillance 25(8) 2020) 23 Jan. 2020 pubmed.ncbi.nlm.nih.gov/31992387/ www.eurosurveillance.org/content/10.2807/1560-7917.ES.2020.25.3.2000045

7. External peer review of the RTPCR test to detect SARS-CoV-2 reveals 10 major scientific flaws at the molecular and methodological level: consequences for false positive results.www.cormandrostenreview.com/report/ 27 Nov. 2020

8. Ealy H, et al. COVID-19 Data Collection, Comorbidity & Federal Law, Science, Public Health Policy & The Law. Vol. 2:4-22, Oct.12, 2020. jdfor2020.com/wp-content/uploads/2020/11/adf864_165a103206974fdbb14ada6bf8af1541.pdf

9. WHO, Coronavirus disease (Covid-19) Serology. Oct. 2020 web.archive.org/web/20201022012953/https://www.who.int/news-room/q-a-detail/coronavirus-disease-covid-19-serology

10. COVID-19: Serology, antibodies and immunity - 13 Nov 2020 web.archive.org/web/20201119212350/https://www.who.int/news-room/q-a-detail/coronavirus-disease-covid-19-serology

11. Event 201 Pandemic Exercise, World Economic Forum. 15 Oct.2019 www.weforum.org/press/2019/10/live-simulation-exercise-to-prepare-public-and-private-leaders-for-pandemic-response

12 Schwab K. *Covid-19: The Great Reset.* Agentur Schweiz, 9 July 2020.

13. Great reset WEF Conference, 3 June 2020. www.weforum.org/agenda/2020/06/now-is-the-time-for-a-great-reset/

14. Supplementary Information with Updates: www.researchgate.net/publication/348894789

15. ourworldindata.org/grapher/daily-covid-cases-deaths?time=2020-01-01..latest (Set the graphic for the US.)

16. ourworldindata.org/grapher/daily-covid-19-tests-smoothed-7-day?time=earliest..latest (Set the graphic for the US.)

17. Lifetime odds of death for selected causes, United States, 2019. www.injuryfacts.nsc.org/all-injuries/preventable-death-overview/odds-of-dying/

18. WHO says COVID-19 pandemic is 'one big wave', not seasonal. www.reuters.com/article/us-health-coronavirus-who-idUSKCN24T16U

19 COVID-19 Doesn't Seem Seasonal, Study Says. www.webmd.com/lung/news/20201014/covid-19-doesnt-seem-seasonal-study-says

20. ourworldindata.org/covid-deaths?country=CAN~FRA~GUF~DEU~GRC~ITA~JPN~ESP~SWE

21. ourworldindata.org/covid-deaths?country=ARG-AUS-CHL-ZAF

22. ourworldindata.org/search?q=Influenza+USA

23. www.ucsf.edu/news/2020/ 09/418606/can-you-tell-if-its-flu-or-covid-19-doctors-say-its-not-so-clear

24. www.medscape.com/viewarticle/924728 (See CDC Jan.2020 archive)

25. Coronavirus Is Bad but US Flu's New Numbers Still Far Worse (3 Feb.2020) www.cdc.gov/flu/weekly/index.htm#S13

26. The missing flu riddle. justthenews.com/politics-policy/coronavirus/influenza-levels-continue-cratering-some-cite-covid-measures-even-covid

27. www.gis.cdc.gov/grasp/fluview/mortality.html

28. www.cdc.gov/flu/weekly/index.htm

29. www.cdc.gov/flu/weekly/weeklyarchives2020-2021/ILI13.html

30. www.cdc.gov/nchs/nvss/vsrr/covid_weekly/index.htm

31. Wilhelm Reich's Bion-Biogenesis Discoveries. youtu.be/-PVnS72IIY8

32. New Images of Novel Coronavirus SARS-CoV-2 Now Available. www.niaid.nih.gov/news-events/novel-coronavirus-sarscov2-images

33. MERS-CoV Images. www.flickr.com/photos/niaid/albums/72157634229836113

34. SARS-CoV-2 Images. www.flickr.com/photos/niaid/albums/72157712914621487

35. Borger P, et al. External peer review of the RTPCR test to detect SARS-CoV-2 reveals 10 major scientific flaws at the molecular and methodological level: consequences for false positive results. www.cormandrostenreview.com/report/

36. Farber C. Ten Fatal Errors: Scientists Attack Paper That Established Global PCR Driven Lockdown. 3 Dec.2020. uncoverdc.com/2020/12/03/ten-fatal-errors-scientists-attack-paper-that-established-global-pcr-driven-lockdown/

37. Farber C. Was the COVID-19 Test Meant to Detect a Virus? 7 April 2020. uncoverdc.com/2020/04/07/was-the-covid-19-test-meant-to-detect-a-virus/

38. Mercola J. COVID-19 Testing Scandal Deepens. 18 Dec.2020. articles.mercola.com/sites/articles/archive/2020/12/18/pcr-test-reliability.aspx

39. High coronavirus positive case rate reveals flaws in Florida Department of Health report. clickorlando.com/news/local/2020/07/15/high-coronavirus-positive-case-rate-reveals-flaws-in-florida-department-of-health-report/

40. Kary Mullis, Nobel Lecture. 8 Dec.1993. www.nobelprize.org/prizes/chemistry/1993/mullis/lecture/

41. WHO Information Notice for IVD Users 2020/05. www.who.int/news/item/20-01-2021-who-information-notice-for-ivd-users-2020-05

42. COVID-19 vaccine breakthrough case investigation: Information for public health, clinical, and reference laboratories. www.cdc.gov/vaccines/covid-19/downloads/Information-for-laboratories-COVID-vaccine-breakthrough-case-investigation.pdf

43. Hospitals get paid more if patients listed as COVID-19, on ventilators. www.usatoday.com/story/news/factcheck/2020/04/24/fact-check-medicare-hospitals-paid-more-covid-19-patients-coronavirus/3000638001/ – Hospital Payments and the COVID-19 Death Count. www.factcheck.org/2020/04/hospital-payments-and-the-covid-19-death-count/

44. Bianchi F, et al. The Long Term Impact of the Covid-19 Unemployment Shock on Life Expectancy and Mortality Rates. Jan.2021. www.nber.org/system/files/working_papers/w28304/w28304.pdf

45. BANNED/CENSORED: www.youtube.com/watch?v=3cjgicrA504

46. Cummins I. Viral Update Dec.7 2020. Europe USA. content.streamhoster.com/file/osom/osom/CumminsViralUpdateDec7thEuropeUSAexplained.mov?dl=1

47. NY Times: Reopening Plans and Mask Mandates for All 50 States. nytimes.com/interactive/2020/us/states-reopen-map-coronavirus.html

48. Published Papers and Data on Lockdown Weak Efficacy – and Lockdown Huge Harms. thefatemperor.com/published-papers-and-data-on-lockdown-weak-efficacy-and-lockdown-huge-harms/ – www.researchgate.net/publication/348894789

49. Collateral Global: Studies: Health. collateralglobal.org

50. Bluestone B, Corporate Flight: Causes and Consequences of Economic Dislocation, Center for Policy Alternatives, 1981. Also: "Is unemployment really as deadly as coronavirus?" nypost.com/2020/04/20/explaining-the-link-between-unemployment-deaths-amid-coronavirus/

51. Amid Rise in Child Self-Harm, Suicidality, Alcohol Deaths Boris Appoints 'Mental Health Ambassador'. www.breitbart.com/europe/2021/02/04/amid-rise-in-child-self-harm-alcohol-deaths-suicidality-boris-johnson-appoints-mental-health-ambassador

52. As the pandemic ushered in isolation and financial hardship, overdose deaths reached new heights. www.statnews.com/2021/02/16/as-pandemic-ushered-in-isolation-financial-hardship-overdose-deaths-reached-new-heights/

53. Harvard Study: An Epidemic of Loneliness Is Spreading Across America. fee.org/articles/harvard-study-an-epidemic-of-loneliness-is-spreading-across-america/

54. Self-harm and substance use disorder among teens rose substantially during pandemic: report. amp.washingtontimes.com/news/2021/mar/3/self-harm-and-substance-use-disorder-among-teens-r/

55. BOMBSHELL: Stats Canada claims lockdowns, not COVID-19, are now driving 'excess deaths'. www.lifesitenews.com/news/bombshell-stats-canada-claims-lockdowns-not-covid-19-are-now-driving-excess-deaths

56. Questions for lockdown apologists. medium.com/@JohnPospichal/questions-for-lockdown-apologists-32a9bbf2e247

57. Study: Dems COVID19 Lockdown Measures Causing Most Deaths. principia-scientific.org/study-covid19-lockdown-measures-causing-most-deaths/

58. COVID-19 (excess) mortalities: viral cause impossible—drugs with key role in about 200,000 extra deaths in Europe and the US alone. realnewsaustralia.com/2020/10/01/covid-19-excess-mortalities-viral-cause-impossible-drugs-with-key-role-in-about-200000-extra-deaths-in-europe-and-the-us-alone/

59. Evaluation of the virulence of SARS-CoV-2 in France, from all-cause mortality 1946-2020. www.researchgate.net/publication/343775235_Evaluation_of_the_virulence_of_SARS-CoV-2_in_France_from_all-cause_mortality_1946-2020

60. Masks, False Safety and Real Dangers. pdmj.org/papers/masks_false_safety_and_real_dangers_part1/ – pdmj.org/papers/masks_false_safety_and_real_dangers_part2/ – pdmj.org/papers/masks_false_safety_and_real_dangers_part3/ – pdmj.org/papers/masks_false_safety_and_real_dangers_part4/

61. ALERT: Meta-Analysis of 65 Studies Reveals Face Masks Induce Mask-Induced Exhaustion Syndrome (MIES). www.greenmedinfo.com/blog/alert-meta-analysis-65-studies-reveals-face-masks-induce-mask-induced-exhaustion-

62. Provisional Death Counts for Coronavirus Disease 2019 (COVID-19) Weekly Updates. www.cdc.gov/nchs/nvss/vsrr/covid_weekly/index.htm

63. Euromomo: Graphs and Maps. www.euromomo.eu/graphs-and-maps

64. Huff, D: *How to Lie With Statistics*, W.W. Norton, 1993.

65. Provisional Death Counts for Coronavirus Disease 2019 (COVID-19) Weekly Updates. www.cdc.gov/nchs/nvss/vsrr/covid_weekly/index.htm

66. Briand G. Covid19 Deaths, a Look at the US Data. www.youtube.com/watch?v=3TKJN61afll

67. Gu Y. A closer look at U.S. deaths due to COVID-19. 22 Nov.2020, CENSORED, with editorial replacing he original. www.jhunewsletter.com/article/2020/11/a-closer-look-at-u-s-deaths-due-to-covid-19

68. Gu Y. A closer look at U.S. deaths due to COVID-19 (original paper, defaced). drive.google.com/file/d/1Tnb1a8TXHj_jJCM2BDfGSriUgdn-2gec/view

69. US deaths in 2020 top 3 million, by far most ever counted. apnews.com/article/us-coronavirus-deaths-top-3-million-e2bc856b6ec45563b84ee2e87ae8d5e7

70. covid.cdc.gov/covid-data-tracker/-cases_casesper100klast7days

71. Johns Hopkins Coronavirus Resource Center. coronavirus.jhu.edu/

72. WHO Coronavirus (COVID-19) Dashboard. Covid19.who.int/

73. Friedlander H, *The Origins of Nazi Genocide: From Euthanasia to the Final Solution*, Univ. North Carolina Press, 1997.

74. Peter Duesberg, *Inventing the AIDS Virus*, Regnery Press, 1985; also *Infectious AIDS: Have We Been Misled?*, North Atlantic Books,1995.

75. James Carter, *Racketeering in Medicine: Suppression of Alternatives*, Hampton Roads, 1992.

76. James DeMeo, "The Suppression of Dissent in Science and Medicine", 2007. www.orgonelab.org/suppression.htm

77. Hydroxychloroquine Has about 90 Percent Chance of Helping COVID-19 Patients. aapsonline.org/hcq-90-percent-chance/ The probabilities of clinical success using hydroxychloroquine with or without azithromycin +/-zinc against the novel betacoronavirus, SARS-CoV-2 drive.google.com/file/d/1w6p_HqRXCrW0_wYNK7m_zpQLbBVYcvVU/view

78. Successful High-Dose Vitamin C Treatment of Patients with Serious and Critical COVID-19 Infection. orthomolecular.org/resources/omns/v16n18.shtml

79. Covid-19 Vulnerability and Vitamin D Deficiency. www.academia.edu/44719317/COVID_19_Vulnerability_and_Vitamin_D_Deficiency

80. Doctors cure 6,000 patients with Covid-19 with Ivermectin. dominicantoday.com/dr/covid-19/2020/09/29/doctors-cure-6000-patients-with-covid-19-with-ivermectin/

81. DeMeo, J: *The Orgone Accumulator Handbook*, Natural Energy Works, 2010.

82. VAERS Data Sets. vaers.hhs.gov/data/datasets.html https://vaersanalysis.info/2021/08/

83. Impact of Covid Vaccinations on Mortality. youtube.com/watch?v=xSrc_s2Gqfw

About the Author

James DeMeo earned his PhD in the field of Geography, with a specialization in Earth and Atmospheric Science. He is author or editor of nine books and around a hundred published research papers in science journals and popular media on environmental-atmospheric issues, biophysical experiments, science history, cross-cultural studies, and health-related subjects. A former university professor, he is today retired doing private research and writing. His scientific works can be reviewed on the ResearchGate.net website.

www.researchgate.net/profile/James-Demeo/research

Other Books by James DeMeo
Available from www.naturalenergyworks.net

The Dynamic Ether of Cosmic Space: Correcting a Major Error in Modern Science

Saharasia: The 4000 BCE Origins of Child Abuse, Sex-Repression, Warfare and Social Violence, In the Deserts of the Old World.

The Orgone Accumulator Handbook: Wilhelm Reich's Life-Energy Discoveries and Healing Tools for the 21st Century, with Construction Plans

In Defense of Wilhelm Reich: Opposing the 80-Years' War of Mainstream Defamatory Slander against One of the 20th Century's Most Brilliant Physicians and Natural Scientists.

Marx Engels Lenin Trotsky: Genocide Quotes. The Hidden History of Communism's Founding Tyrants, in their Own Words.

Preliminary Analysis of Changes in Kansas Weather Coincidental to Experimental Operations with a Reich Cloudbuster: From a 1979 Research Project, reprinted 2010.

(as Editor and Contributor) *Heretic's Notebook: Emotions, Protocells, Ether-Drift and Cosmic Life-Energy, with New Research Supporting Wilhelm Reich.*

(as Editor and Contributor) *On Wilhelm Reich and Orgonomy.*

(as Co-Editor and Contributor) *Nach Reich: Neue Forschungen zur Orgonomie: Sexualökonomie, Die Entdeckung der Orgonenergie.*

For new findings and evidence relevant to this book,
see the "Supplemental Information" update page here:
www.researchgate.net/publication/348894789
Or, check out Dr. DeMeo's informative Facebook page
(assuming it has not yet been censored and erased!)
https://www.facebook.com/jamesdemeophd

To get on James DeMeo's private
Occasional Newsletter **mailing list:**
lp.constantcontactpages.com/su/hozrK9M

**James DeMeo's research is privately funded,
your support is needed and greatly appreciated:**
www.orgonelab.org/donate

www.ingramcontent.com/pod-product-compliance
Lightning Source LLC
Chambersburg PA
CBHW080058280326
41934CB00014B/3363